Rapid health assessment protocols for emergencies

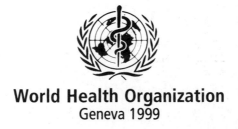

World Health Organization
Geneva 1999

WHO Library Cataloguing in Publication Data

Rapid health assessment protocols for emergencies.

1. Epidemiologic methods 2. Emergencies 3. Disease outbreaks 4. Health services needs and demand 5. Health status 6. Guidelines

ISBN 92 4 154515 1   (NLM Classification: WA 950)

Typeset in Hong Kong
Printed in England
97/11693 — Best Set/Clays — 7500

Contents

Preface

The initial phase of a major emergency is crucial for the survival of victims and for determining the future path of assistance to the stricken community. Many organizations from within and outside the affected country send teams to assess the emergency situation and determine the kind of response required to relieve human suffering. The absence of a common, standardized technical tool for damage and needs assessment in this initial phase may result in contradictory information being channelled to national and international humanitarian agencies. Consequently, the response may be one that fails to meet actual needs, aggravating rather than improving the emergency situation.

To address this gap, this publication brings together, in one volume, 10 protocols designed to help those involved in the rapid assessment determine the immediate and potential health impact of a broad range of emergencies and assist in planning appropriate responses.

The original protocols were the joint effort of three WHO Collaborating Centres for Emergency Preparedness and Response: the Centre for Research on the Epidemiology of Disasters, Brussels, Belgium; the Centers for Disease Control and Prevention, Atlanta, Georgia, USA; and the National Public Health Institute, Department of Environmental Hygiene and Toxicology, Kuopio, Finland. WHO distributed the draft protocols to Member States, the six WHO regional offices, and other WHO partners, including nongovernmental organizations, for extensive field-testing. On the basis of their written comments, the protocols were subsequently reviewed and updated by experts from intergovernmental and nongovernmental organizations with broad experience in the field of emergency management.

This series of protocols is meant to be used as a complete unit; the introduction deals with the basic elements of rapid health assessment, while the subsequent protocols cover specific types of emergencies. Certain topics, common to more than one type of emergency, are covered in only one protocol and cross-referenced to reduce redundancy.

Rapid health assessment is a complex task fraught with difficulties and one that carries heavy responsibilities. Therefore, whenever possible, it should be undertaken only by teams of well qualified and experienced specialists. Nevertheless, there are circumstances in which a life-saving response cannot wait while an expert team is assembled, and key information must be gathered as early as possible. For this reason, the protocols provide background information, so that they may assist general health personnel identify priorities in emergencies and respond accordingly.

The protocols are also intended for personnel and organizations who may not conduct the assessment but have responsibility for emergency preparedness and response, such as ministries of health. They can be used to train emergency workers prior to emergencies, to demonstrate how rapid assessment can be integrated into multisectoral emergency preparedness, and to show how information collected through the assessments can be employed for effective emergency response.

Finally, while the protocols focus on health, they are meant to be used within the context of a larger assessment of the status and emergency needs of all aspects of a community. To be effective, emergency preparedness must be institutionalized at every level of management in countries vulnerable to major emergencies. This institutionalization comprises policy development, vulnerability assessment, emergency planning, developing information and resource management systems, training and education, and monitoring and evaluation. All major development activities should include a component of emergency preparedness to reduce the harm caused by emergencies. Without this component, thousands of people's lives are at risk and sustainable development is in jeopardy.

No one sector of a country or community is wholly responsible for every aspect of an emergency. However, each sector and organization should plan assessment activities, train personnel in assessment techniques, and practise these techniques with other sectors and organizations. Rapid assessment should be the joint activity of all humanitarian agencies so that they may provide definitive information to response and recovery decision-makers. The working partnerships and open communication that contribute to emergency preparedness lay the foundation for effective coordination and cooperation in times of actual emergencies.

WHO wishes to acknowledge the contributions of the following to the review and finalization of the protocols: Dr V. Brown, Médecins Sans Frontières/Epicentre; Dr R. Coninx, International Committee of the Red Cross; Dr M. Dualeh, Office of the United Nations High Commissioner for Refugees; Mr T. Foster, Registered Engineers for Disaster Relief; Mr A. Mourey, International Committee of the Red Cross; Dr H. Sandbladh, International Federation of Red Cross and Red Crescent Societies; and Dr B. Woodruff, Centers for Disease Control and Prevention. In addition, the following WHO personnel participated in updating the technical content of the protocols: Ms M. Anker, Division of Emerging and other Communicable Diseases Surveillance and Control; Dr K. Bailey, formerly of the Division of Food and Nutrition; Dr S. Ben Yahmed, formerly of the Division of Emergency and Humanitarian Action; Mr H. Dixon, formerly of the Division of Health Situation and Trend Assessment; Ms H. Hailemeskal, formerly of the Division of Emergency and Humanitarian Action; Mr P. Koob (editorial assistance), formerly of the Division of Emergency and Humanitarian Action; Dr J. Le Duc, formerly of the Division of Emerging and other Communicable Diseases Surveillance and Control; Dr A. Loretti, Panafrican Emergency Training Centre, Addis Ababa; Dr K. Nguyen, formerly of the Division of Emerging and other Communicable Diseases Surveillance and Control; Ms M. Petevi, Division of Mental Health and Prevention of Substance Abuse; Dr M. Santamaria, Division of Emerging and other Communicable Diseases Surveillance and Control; Mr M. Szczeniowski, Division of Emerging and other Communicable Diseases Surveillance and Control; and Dr E. Tikhomirov, Division of Emerging and other Communicable Diseases Surveillance and Control.

Chapter 1
Rapid health assessment

Purpose

In emergency management, assessment means collecting subjective and objective information in order to measure damage and identify those basic needs of the affected population that require immediate response. The assessment is always meant to be rapid, as it must be performed in limited time, during or in the immediate aftermath of an emergency.

At the onset of a crisis, rapid assessment information will be used to recognize and quantify the emergency, and to readjust strategies and plans accordingly. Once a programme of assistance is under way, periodic assessments will assist evaluation of the effectiveness of response and recovery. In a wider perspective, rapid assessment will produce information for financial and political advocacy, public information, press releases, and case studies.

The information produced by the assessment is both an asset and a commodity. It must be used for vital decision-making, and for feedback along the different levels of the health sector. But this information can also be marketed to other sectors. Mutual exchange of information is the first step in effective coordination, and being recognized as a reliable source of information is the best way for an organization to assert its claim to a coordinating role.

The purpose of a rapid assessment is to:

— confirm the emergency;
— describe the type, impact and possible evolution of the emergency;
— measure its present and potential health impact;
— assess the adequacy of existing response capacity and immediate additional needs; and
— recommend priority action for immediate response.

Preparedness

If the rapid assessment is to be useful for guiding emergency health response, it must be clear in advance which individuals make the decisions on emergency interventions because they must receive the information and recommendations made by the rapid assessment team. Moreover, it is essential that responsibilities for each particular emergency health action are clearly defined at national, regional, and local levels. Ideally, the rapid assessment should be conducted as the cooperative effort of all organizations with responsibilities for emergency response.

While it is impossible to plan for all potential emergencies, the challenge for all health programmes is how best to make emergency preparedness a part of their current activities, to both strengthen existing services and prepare for emergency response. Emergency preparedness includes:

— policy development for preparedness, response and recovery;
— vulnerability assessment;
— emergency planning;
— training and education; and
— monitoring and evaluation.

Emergency plans should be prepared by the ministry of health for all anticipated emergencies. These plans should include a description of:

— management structure (emergency powers, control, command, communication, emergency coordination centres, and post-emergency review);
— organization roles (description by role, description by organization, description by sector and emergency operation centres);
— information management (alerting, emergency assessment, information processing, public information, reporting, and translation and interpreting);
— resource management (resource coordination, administration, financial procedures, external assistance);
— summary of vulnerability assessment;
— maps; and
— emergency contacts.

Provisions for the assessment should be part of these emergency plans. There should be clear mechanisms in place for incorporating the assessment findings in emergency decision-making.

Emergency health response does not always need to wait for the collection of data. Experience has shown that emergencies have specific, predictable patterns of impact on public health. Selected health responses can and should be planned in advance, ready to be carried out without awaiting the results of rapid health assessment.

An example of this is the higher risk of measles epidemics among children in displaced populations living in camps. In countries at increased risk of internal or cross-border displacements, the national programme of immunization should include strategies to prevent such outbreaks as part of preparedness planning. Another example applies to countries at increased risk of sudden-impact emergencies such as earthquakes: routine hospital management in these areas must include formulating mass casualty plans and holding regular emergency practice drills. In communities with chemical plants, formulating in advance standard treatment guidelines for chemical exposure makes prompt case management possible, should a chemical incident occur.

Preparedness checklist

These questions can be adapted for specific types of health emergencies. They can also provide a focus for health preparedness activities at regional, district, and community levels.

1. Is there a national health policy regarding emergency preparedness, response, and recovery? Is the policy being implemented?
2. Is there a person within the ministry of health in charge of promoting, developing, and coordinating emergency preparedness, response, and recovery activities?
3. What coordination in emergency preparedness activities exists between the health sector, civil defence, and key ministries (such as the ministry of the interior and the ministry of agriculture)?
4. What joint activities in emergency preparedness, response, and recovery are undertaken between the ministry of health, United Nations organizations, and nongovernmental organizations (NGOs)?
5. Are there operational plans for health response to natural, man-made or other emergencies?
6. Have mass casualty management plans been developed (both pre-hospital and hospital) at national level as well as for individual hospitals?
7. What health and nutrition surveillance measures have been taken for the early detection of health emergencies (high-risk seasons, geographical areas identified; early warning procedures in place; national reference laboratory established; surveillance system established and working)?
8. What preparedness steps have been taken by environmental health services?
9. Have facilities and areas been identified and designated as temporary settlements in the event of emergencies? What provisions have been made for health care? (Include details such as general or special health services, staffing, supplies, water, and sanitation.)
10. What training activities are devoted to emergency preparedness, response, and recovery in the health sector (at national, regional, and district levels) and what organizations are involved?
11. What resources are available to facilitate a rapid health response (e.g. an organized communications centre in the ministry of health, emergency budget, access to transport, and emergency medical supplies)?
12. Is there a system for updating information on the key human and material resources needed for an emergency health response (e.g. updated inventories of essential drugs, and four-wheel-drive vehicles)?
13. What opportunities exist to test emergency plans through, for example, simulation exercises and drills?

Organizational preparedness

The measures listed below are of particular concern to managers within the ministry of health. Such measures are essential components of health emergency preparedness and should be reflected in all the ministry's technical programmes.

The following structures for emergency health response should be in place:

— a position in the ministry of health with overall authority and responsibility for emergency health response;
— executive structures at all levels, with clear responsibilities for emergency health response (e.g. emergency health committees at community, district, regional, and central levels);
— a clear chain of command from central to peripheral levels for emergency health management;
— working links at all levels between the ministry of health, national emergency response and recovery organizations, the World Health Organization (WHO), the United Nations Children's Fund (UNICEF), the United Nations High Commissioner for Refugees (UNHCR), the United Nations Development Programme (UNDP), the World Food Programme (WFP), NGOs, and bilateral and intergovernmental organizations involved in health and nutrition; and
— coordination with other sectors, such as health, lifelines, transport, police and investigation, and social welfare.

Prepare emergency plans for anticipated emergencies

It is important to identify emergencies likely to occur at national and subnational levels, and their probable health consequences. Simple emergency plans, prepared and approved within the ministry of health, should outline the administrative and technical responsibilities and procedures necessary for a timely response. These plans and procedures should then be distributed to the relevant organizations involved in emergency response.

Existing information and experience gained in past emergencies are useful in setting priorities. The following questions should be considered:

• Where were the high-risk areas in past health emergencies? Who are the populations at risk? Based on experience, when are the high-risk seasons?
• What is the likely health impact of a flood or epidemic of meningitis? (Consider the number of cases, hospital admissions, and deaths.)

Compile and update information for prompt response

• Establish procedures for communicating early signs of possible emergencies between health authorities, key ministries, national emergency response organizations, international organizations, and NGOs so that a prompt alert is signaled.
• Keep updated lists and maps of health facilities, with information on bed capacity and specialist services available.
• Keep an updated inventory of NGOs working in health in the country, and their areas of expertise and experience in emergencies.
• In areas at high risk for health emergencies, have detailed maps available showing airfields, access roads, health facilities, and major water sources.

Clarify areas of responsibility and accountability

• Clarify who is responsible for emergency health action at each administrative level.

- Determine which organization is responsible for:
  - multi-organization coordination in an emergency (lead agency for the rapid assessment);
  - clearance, storage, and transport of emergency items;
  - directing technical health response; and
  - other critical activities such as travel clearances.

Standardize approaches to international health assistance
- Clarify reporting channels or lines of accountability for international organizations and NGOs.
- Develop standard procedures for requesting external health assistance.
- Establish standard working procedures for the importation and expedited clearance of emergency health items and drugs.

Anticipate needs for budget, transport, and communications
- Establish procedures for accessing funds and resources in health emergencies.
- Identify emergency options for rapid surface and air transport of personnel and emergency health items.
- Set up procedures for rapid collection, transport, and analysis of laboratory specimens.
- Establish procedures for emergency communication with peripheral areas.

Deal with the technical aspects
Plans of action should be developed for the early detection of and response to anticipated health emergencies. A useful starting point is to review and map existing data on past emergencies to identify areas of greatest risk, and assess local response capacity. The rapid health assessment team or person should ask people from the ministry of health or provincial or district health services the following questions:

- What is the distribution of facilities, number of beds, number of specialist services, and seasonal access to the area and facilities?
- How many health workers are there in the area and what is their level of experience?
- What are the likely effects of specific emergencies on health services in the areas identified as high risk (e.g. consider the number of admissions and the outpatient attendance)?
- What is needed for a prompt emergency response (e.g. hospital staff trained in mass casualty management, experienced epidemiologist, improved radio communication, and training of clinicians for better diagnosis)?
- Where are the gaps (in technical expertise, material supplies, emergency logistics, communication, and managerial skills)?

Establish early warning procedures
- Define the early signs that would signal an "emergency alert". Can or could they be detected early through improved surveillance and reporting?
- Develop guidelines to help health personnel at all levels recognize and report these signs.

- Intensify surveillance for specific epidemic diseases during high-risk transmission periods.

Preparedness for rapid assessment

An important function of emergency planning is to identify in advance those warning signals which indicate that a rapid health assessment is needed. Alerts for these signals should also be determined, as shown in Table 1.

These alerts should be related to local conditions and expected seasonal variations. Ideally they will be triggered by ongoing activities such as epidemiological and nutritional surveillance.

Although all of the following seven measures are not always feasible, they are very desirable if the assessment is to be carried out rapidly.

1. Lines of authority within the ministry of health should be defined and clearly stated.
2. Organizational networks and partnerships should be maintained for mobilizing personnel and resources for the rapid assessment.
3. National, subnational, and district maps of high-risk areas, showing settlements, water sources, main transport routes, and health facilities, should be developed, kept updated, and made easily available.
4. Data collection forms, specimen containers, and other items essential for specific types of field assessments should be kept at the national and subnational levels.
5. Reference laboratories and special shipment procedures for rapid analysis of specimens should be identified in advance.
6. Communication channels between the assessment team, local authorities, decision-makers, and participating organizations should be agreed upon and kept open.
7. Qualified personnel should be identified in advance for rapid health assessment in specific types of emergencies.

Preparedness provides an opportunity to identify local skilled individuals as potential assessors in different types of emergencies, and to highlight gaps in technical expertise in advance. Although a rapid health assessment is usually best undertaken by a team, the composition of the group will vary according to the type of emergency.

Table 1. Warning signals of emergencies

Warning signal	Alert
An increase in hospitals reporting cases of meningococcal meningitis	Give alert for a meningitis outbreak
Above-expected seasonal levels of the disease in one district	
Rising prices of staple cereals, and migration of people into an area that is expected to have a major crop failure at harvest time	Give famine alert
Increasing hospital admissions with signs of irritation of the eyes, skin, and mucous membranes in a community near a chemical plant	Give alert for a chemical accident

For instance, it is more important that a nutritionist participate in assessing a refugee influx than a meningitis outbreak. However, an individual skilled in epidemiology or public health should be a member of every assessment team.

Planning the assessment

This section contains information on: time and distance factors in emergencies, final preparations, the assessment itself, the best working practices, and common sources of error.

The seven preparedness measures listed in the previous section can also serve as a checklist for planning a rapid health assessment when an emergency is reported or rumoured.

Considering time and distance factors

Rapid assessment time-frame requirements and opportunities vary with the type of event and the accessibility of the affected area. In general, the following holds true:

- Rapid-onset emergencies, such as earthquakes and chemical accidents, require the most immediate assessment, in a matter of hours after the impact.
- Epidemics, floods and sudden displacements of population should be assessed at the latest within two to four days.
- In the case of suspected famine, where the onset is usually slower and an adequate investigation requires sampling the population, the assessment may take somewhat longer.
- In some situations, logistic or security considerations (e.g. in complex emergencies) may reduce the time available for conducting the assessment at field level to a few hours.

Distance or difficult access to the affected area, or both, can delay the initial assessment. If several areas have been affected, or the emergency is thought to have had widespread impact, several small assessment teams may be needed. In almost all situations, the initial rapid assessment should be followed by a more thorough and focused one. In particular, when the effectiveness of emergency response is being evaluated, it is necessary to collect baseline information through surveys that use probability sampling of the population.

Making the final preparations

The final preparations include: determining what information to gather, coordinating different organizations, selecting team members, identifying the team leader and assigning tasks, and making administrative arrangements.

Determining what information to gather

The two most important criteria for deciding what information to collect in a rapid assessment are its usefulness for timely decision-making and its public health importance.

Coordinating different organizations

Members of the rapid health assessment team should contact as many as possible of the organizations delivering emergency response, to coordinate activities and avoid duplicating efforts. Coordination and pooling of resources can produce a more complete and rapid assessment.

Selecting team members

The rapid health assessment should be performed by a multidisciplinary team of qualified personnel, representing an appropriate range of expertise. For example, a team to assess the health needs of a refugee population should include an individual from each of the following fields: public health and epidemiology, nutrition, logistics, and environmental health.

The following criteria should be taken into account in selecting team members:

— familiarity with the region or population affected;
— knowledge of and experience with the type of emergency being assessed;
— personal qualities, such as endurance, motivation, and personal health, the capacity for teamwork, and local acceptability for team members recruited abroad;
— analytical skills, particularly the ability to see trends and patterns; and
— the capacity to make correct decisions in unstructured situations on the basis of relatively sparse data.

Identifying the team leader and assigning tasks

One team leader must be identified to coordinate technical preparations for the field assessment, such as delegating responsibilities among members, ensuring consistency in approach and use of questionnaires, and preparing laboratory supplies and other equipment.

Making administrative arrangements

These include:

— obtaining travel and security clearances;
— organizing transportation and other logistics (e.g. vehicles, fuel, and, in some cases, camping equipment, food, and beverages);
— setting up the communications system and informing the authorities in the affected area of the assessment's timetable;
— organizing other equipment, such as computers, height boards, scales, and checklists; and
— ensuring safety and security of team members from violence, infection or other hazards in the emergency-affected area.

Conducting the assessment

The steps for carrying out the assessment are: collecting data, analysing them, presenting results and conclusions, and monitoring.

Always take into consideration the following questions:

- How feasible is it to collect this information, given available personnel and resources?
- Is it worth the cost?
- How reliably do the data reflect the situation of the entire population affected by the emergency, i.e. how representative are they?

Collecting the data

Emergencies are often chaotic, and data collection during a rapid health assessment may not proceed in a step-by-step, logical fashion. Yet the plan for data collection and analysis must be systematic. In addition, the limitations of the various sources of information must be borne in mind during data collection and analysis. There are four main methods of collecting data:

— review of existing information;
— visual inspection of the affected area;
— interviews with key informants; and
— rapid surveys.

Review of existing information

Review baseline health and other information at national and regional levels from government, international, bilateral, and NGO sources about the following:

— the geographical and environmental characteristics of the affected area;
— administrative and political divisions of the affected area;
— the size, composition, and prior health and nutritional condition of the population affected by the emergency;
— health services and programmes functioning before the emergency; and
— resources already allocated, procured or requested for the emergency response operation.

Even official data sources are subject to limitations. For example, census data may underestimate certain subgroups or the population as a whole. In addition, morbidity surveillance data may represent an incomplete picture because diseases are routinely under-reported and the extent of under-reporting often varies.

Visual inspection of the affected area

When travel is undertaken by air, useful preliminary observations of the affected area can be made before landing. These may include a gross estimate of the extent of the disaster-affected area (e.g. the extent of flooding or of storm damage), mass population movements, condition of infrastructure (e.g. roads and railways), and of the environment.

A walk through the emergency-affected area may give you a general idea of the adequacy of shelter, food availability, environmental factors (such as drainage and vector breeding), other potential hazards, and the status of the population. The age and sex distribution and size of the population should be estimated.

During the observation, the affected area should be roughly mapped. Such maps should indicate the extent of the area affected, the distribution of the population, and the location of resources, including medical facilities, water sources, food distribution points, and temporary shelters.

Even careful observation may result in a biased impression. If the area visited is more or less severely hit than the rest, the observer may think the overall condition of the entire affected area is better or worse than it is. In addition, the most severely affected persons are often the least visible; injured or sick persons are more likely to be inside shelters and less accessible to visitors.

Interviewing key informants

Conduct interviews with key personnel in the area and with persons from every sector of the affected population:

- clan, village, and community leaders;
- area administrators or other government officials, teachers;
- health workers (including traditional birth attendants and healers);
- personnel from local and international emergency response organizations, including United Nations bodies working in the area; and
- individuals in the affected population.

The information collected from these interviews should include:

- the interviewees' perception of the event (cause and dynamics);
- pre-emergency conditions in the affected area;
- geographical distribution and size of the affected population;
- age and sex distribution of the population and average household size;
- adequacy of security and prevalence of violence;
- current morbidity and death rates and causes;
- current food supplies, recent food distribution, and future food needs;
- current supply and quality of water;
- current adequacy of sanitation;
- other priority needs of the affected population, such as shelter and clothing;
- current status of transport, fuel, communication, and other logistic necessities; and
- current resources available in the affected community, including medical equipment, drugs, and personnel.

Concerns expressed by the people interviewed can be further investigated during the rapid health assessment. For example, if health workers report an outbreak of cholera in the emergency-affected area, this should be confirmed or refuted immediately by the assessment team.

The interview with key personnel should be used for planning the establishment of a surveillance system monitoring morbidity, mortality, and nutritional status.

Assessment personnel should always keep in mind that information derived from interviews is coloured by the interviewees' perceptions. These perceptions are subject to the same biases mentioned above regarding visits to the affected area. Moreover, informants may intentionally exaggerate the extent of damage, injury or illness to solicit emergency assistance for the population they represent.

Rapid surveys

Because surveys take more time and resources, they should be reserved for data which are essential but may not be available from other sources. Such data could include:

— sex and age distribution of the affected population;
— average family size;
— number of persons in vulnerable groups, such as unaccompanied children, single women, households headed by women, and destitute elders;
— recent death rates;
— recent rates of health conditions that are specific to the type of emergency, such as diarrhoea, traumatic injuries, burns, and respiratory distress;
— nutritional status;
— vaccination coverage among children;
— state of housing; and
— access to health care, food, water, and shelter.

For a more complete description of survey techniques for rapid health assessment, see Annex 1.

Analysing the data

The data collected during the rapid assessment must be analysed quickly and thoroughly, and the results made available to decision-makers as soon as possible to derive the greatest benefit from the information.

The analysis should use standard techniques to ensure its comparability to assessments conducted in other situations, and to subsequent assessments that will be carried out during the current emergency. For example, standard case definitions for diseases should be used.

The analysis should be as specific as possible to ensure the best targeting for interventions. Data should be disaggregated and treated separately, according to administrative area, period, and type of population, to get specific estimates. The sources of data should always be specified, and an attempt made to assess their reliability.

Presenting results and conclusions

The presentation of the results and conclusions of the rapid assessment should have the following characteristics.

• It should be clear. Decision-makers or staff of local, national, and international organizations whose action depends on the results of the rapid assessment may have little training in interpreting health and epidemiological data. User-friendly language should be used; graphs can help make complex data and trends more easily understood.
• It should be standardized. The results should be presented in widely recognized formats so that they can be compared with other assessments.

For example, the prevalence of moderate and severe malnutrition should be expressed as a percentage of the target population. In an emergency due to sudden population displacement, mortality should be calculated as the number of deaths per 10 000 people per day.

- It should give clear indication of the highest priority needs and how to address them. Chronic or pre-existing conditions and needs should be distinguished from the new ones related to the emergency. The members of the rapid assessment team should arrive at clear recommendations for implementing organizations. For a suggested standard report format, see page 85.
- It should be widely distributed. Copies of the report should be distributed to all organizations involved in the emergency response operations.

Monitoring

The rapid health assessment should be only the first step in collecting data. Ongoing data collection is necessary to evaluate the effect of health programmes implemented before or as a result of the rapid assessment. For example, after recent death or morbidity rates are calculated from data derived from a survey conducted during the rapid assessment, a surveillance system should be established, or reestablished, to monitor future trends.

Developing the best working practices

Ensuring good team work

- International personnel should ensure that national staff participate in the assessment. Likewise, national personnel should include local or district staff in the exercise.
- At field level, introduce yourself and outline quickly the objectives and the method of the assessment. Do not intimidate your interlocutors with unheard-of United Nations or NGO names and abbreviations. Carry visiting cards.
- Explain what you are doing and why. The best way not to be an "emergency tourist" is to discuss on the spot your preliminary conclusions and give new ideas and hints on what you are going to do with the information gathered. Leave behind a copy of your questionnaire as a contribution or as a start-up for a local information system.
- If part of a multisectoral or multi-organizational team:
  — work together at developing and readjusting case definitions and methods;
  — share your questionnaire forms and familiarize yourself with those of other sectors (if the team has to split up to cover more ground in less time, any member should be able to collect data on any issue); and
  — reserve half an hour every day for mutual debriefing.

Making the best of available information

- In emergencies, hard data may appear unattainable. But cross-matching data can provide an idea of the overall quality of information. Likewise, by contacting as many sources as possible, you may be able to put together an unexpected quantity of secondary data.

- The lack (or poor quality) of information is in itself information. A sector or area that does not report is one that has a problem.
- Inaccessibility may be the greatest constraint to the assessment. Try to quantify how much of the situation is actually reflected by your data, defining the accessible areas, the "grey zones" and the "black holes" on the map.
- The situation may change quickly. Collect the most recent data and continue monitoring after the rapid assessment. Circulate and discuss preliminary conclusions while processing the final report.
- Keep a record of geographical distances between major points, such as organizations' offices, warehouses, and water sources. This will assist in planning emergency response.
- Carry with you reference values (e.g. cut-off values for death rates and standard nutritional requirements) for on-the-spot evaluation and preliminary planning. (Annex 2 carries a list of reference values that have proved useful in Africa and that can be adapted for other regions.)
- Keep separate notes of factual observations and personal impressions; if you have a personal computer, record them daily.

Being a good citizen
- Before leaving the capital or provincial headquarters, offer to carry mail, newspapers, or a reasonable amount of supplies to the field stations; carry with you some small luxury, such as fruit or a newspaper, to leave behind.
- Realize that emergency response field-workers labour under heavy workloads and difficult living conditions and that they will stay behind, while you come and go. Pose your questions in a non-threatening way, show appreciation for the good being done, and express criticism constructively.
- If, in the field, you find relevant documents (e.g. registers and reports), copy the information. *Never take away the originals with you.*
- Be ready to assist in medical evacuations from the field, making room for sick or wounded in your vehicle or plane.

Reviewing common sources of error
Common sources of error may be logistic, organizational, or technical.

Logistic
- Transportation and fuel are insufficient for the assessment.
- Communications between field, regional, and national levels are inadequate: the authorities in charge of the area(s) targeted for assessment are not informed on time and are not ready to assist the team.

Organizational
- A lead organization is not designated, the responsibilities of the various organizations are not well defined, and a team leader is not appointed.
- Key decision-makers and potential donors are either not informed that an assessment is being undertaken, or feel pressured to respond to political demands before the findings are known — resulting in inappropriate assistance.

- The assessment is conducted too late or it takes too long.
- Information is collected that is not needed for the planning of the emergency response.

Technical
- Specialists with appropriate skills and experience are not involved in the assessment.
- Programmes that could be implemented immediately, on the basis of past experience, are unnecessarily delayed until the assessment is complete.
- Assessment conclusions are based on data that do not represent the true needs of the affected population (e.g. from non-representative surveys).
- Information received from field-workers and official interviews is taken at face value, without cross-checking all sources.
- A surveillance system is developed too slowly, thus preventing monitoring and evaluation of the emergency response programme.

Presenting the results of the assessment

The following format can be adapted for presenting the results of the assessment in different situations.

- Reason for emergency (type of actual or imminent hazard):
  — onset and evolution;
  — additional hazards.
- Description of the affected area (add at least a sketch map).
- Description of the affected population:
  — number, estimated breakdown by age, sex, and special risk or vulnerability factors;
  — estimated total number of deaths and injuries.
- Impact, in terms of mortality and morbidity:
  — daily crude mortality (number of deaths for the day per 10000 population);
  — other indicators, such as malnutrition rates, losses in vital infrastructures, financial losses and other socioeconomic data can be used.
- Existing response capacity (in terms of human and material resources):
  — local, subnational, and national capacity;
  — international organizations (bilateral, nongovernmental, and intergovernmental);
  — overall authority and national focal point;
  — distribution of tasks and responsibilities;
  — coordination mechanisms;
  — logistics, communications, and administrative support.
- Additional requirements:
  — immediate vital needs of the affected populations;
  — immediate and medium-term needs for national capacity-building;
  — implementation, monitoring, and evaluation mechanisms.

Whenever possible, this section should include medium-term and long-term outlines for rehabilitation and vulnerability reduction.

- Recommendations. Indicate the following:
  - priority actions by projects;
  - responsible office (national focal point and national and international partners);
  - time frame;
  - breakdown of requirements by projects (estimated costs).

An annex should illustrate the timetable of the assessment, give a summary of the methods used and list the sources. It will also include maps and a copy of the questionnaires used and the background documents that may have been collected in the field.

Chapter 2

Epidemics of infectious origin

Purpose of assessment

Infectious diseases of many kinds are present in all human populations. Each population has an expected level of occurrence of each type of disease, and increases in these levels can result in an outbreak, epidemic or epidemic emergency.

Epidemics may occur as the result of an emergency or as an emergency in their own right. The potential risk of an epidemic may be influenced by a number of conditions, including:

— pre-existing disease levels, degree of immunity, and nutritional status;
— environmental change;
— changes in population density and movement of populations;
— disruption of water and sewage services; and
— disruption of basic health services.

An early response to an outbreak or threatened epidemic will often significantly reduce mortality and morbidity in the affected population and limit the spread of the disease to other populations. Rapid health assessment is a key part of such an early response.

The purpose of this rapid assessment is to:

— confirm the threat or existence of an actual epidemic;
— assess its health and socioeconomic impact and likely evolution; and
— assess local response capacity and identify the most effective control measures to minimize the epidemic's effects.

Table 2 gives examples of epidemic disease emergencies.

Preparedness

In dealing with epidemics, the steps below must be carried out, along with the seven preparedness measures listed in Chapter 1, so that the assessment can be rapid.

• Make preliminary preparations for rapid collection and shipment of specimens to reference laboratories.
• Assemble standard data collection forms, specimen containers, slides, and other laboratory supplies for the epidemic diseases that are likely to occur.

- Stock the necessary protective clothing and equipment against potential communicable diseases associated with high mortality.
- Clarify procedures for national and international disease reporting.

Team members should be technically competent to assess the suspected disease both clinically and epidemiologically, and knowledgeable about other diseases possibly involved. Optimally, they should have received training in rapid epidemic assessment, or have prior experience in outbreak investigation.

Conducting the assessment

The decision to mount an epidemic emergency response and the extent of this effort are determined by:

— the seriousness of its actual or potential health impact on the population; and
— the ability of the local health services to respond.

These two factors should be given priority during the assessment.

The five most important questions to take into account are:

- What is the geographical distribution of cases and how many people are at risk?
- How serious is the clinical course of the disease?
- Is the epidemic spreading?
- What could be possible mode(s) of transmission?
- Can local health services cope?

The rapid assessment consists of confirming the existence of an epidemic, assessing its impact on health, and assessing the existing response capacity and additional immediate needs.

Confirming the existence of an epidemic

The first alert or rumour that an epidemic emergency is occurring may come from a wide range of sources, such as local government personnel, citizens, the press, and health care workers. Some sources are not always reliable. A rapid site visit is necessary to verify or refute these initial reports.

To confirm the existence of an epidemic, the diagnosis must be confirmed, an initial case definition established, and the increase in cases verified.

Confirm the diagnosis
This should be carried out by:

— clinical examination of a sample of patients by an expert;
— confirmation of the validity of any supporting laboratory test; and
— collection and testing of additional specimens in a reference laboratory.

Table 2. **Examples of emergencies related to epidemics or potential epidemics**

Disease	In non-endemic areas	In endemic areas
Cholera	One confirmed indigenous case.	Significant increase in incidence over and above what is normal for the season, particularly if multifocal and accompanied by deaths in children less than 10 years old.
Giardiasis	A cluster of cases in a group of tourists returning from an endemic area.	A discrete increase in incidence linked to a specific place.
Malaria	A cluster of cases, with an increase in incidence in a defined geographical area.	Rarely an emergency; increased incidence requires programme strengthening.
Meningococcal meningitis	A 3- to 4-fold increase in cases compared with a similar time period in previous years may indicate an epidemic, as may a doubling of meningitis cases from one week to the next for a period of three weeks.	For countries with high rates of endemic meningitis, such as those within the traditional meningitis belt, a rate of 15 cases per 100 000 per week in a given area, averaged over two consecutive weeks, appears to be a sensitive and specific predictor of epidemic disease in this area.
Plague	One confirmed case.	(a) A cluster of cases apparently linked by domestic rodent or respiratory transmission, or (b) a rodent epizootic.
Rabies	One confirmed case of animal rabies in a previously rabies-free country.	Significant increase in animal and human cases.
Salmonellosis	Not applicable.	A large cluster of cases in a limited area, with a single or predominant serotype, or a significant number of cases occurring in multiple foci apparently related by a common source (not forgetting that several countries may be involved).

Smallpox	Any strongly suspected case. The WHO smallpox eradication campaign succeeded in eliminating the disease in 1980; vigilant surveillance of pox-like diseases (e.g. varicella, monkeypox) is maintained during the post-eradication era.	Not applicable.
Typhus fever due to *Rickettsia prowazekii*	One confirmed case in a louse-infested, non-immune population.	Significant increase in the number of cases in a limited period of time.
Viral encephalitis, mosquito-borne	Cluster of time- and space-related cases in a non-immune population (a single case should be regarded as a warning).	Significant increase in the number of cases with a single identified etiological agent, in a limited period of time.
Viral haemorrhagic fever	One confirmed indigenous or imported case with an etiological agent with which person-to-person transmission may occur.	Significant increase in the number of cases with a single identified etiological agent, in a limited period of time.
Yellow fever	One confirmed case in a community with a non-immune human population and an adequate vector population.	Significant increase in the number of cases in a limited period of time.

Sources:
1. *Public health action in emergencies. caused by epidemics.* Geneva, World Health Organization, 1986.
2. *Control of epidemic meningococcal disease: WHO practical guidelines.* Lyon, Fondation Marcel Merieux, 1995.

Establish an initial case definition

Establish a working case definition after examining patients, meeting with local health workers, and reviewing hospital records. This is essential for guiding early field investigations and identifying cases.

For example, an initial case definition in an outbreak of food-borne disease identified as a "dysentery-like" syndrome was: "a person having bloody diarrhoea and one or more of the following signs and symptoms: fever, nausea, vomiting, abdominal cramps, and tenesmus."

Confirm the increase in the number of cases

Look at local records and compare the current incidence of disease to historical levels in the same population. Make sure that the increase in cases is not spurious, owing to an increased detection of a constant number of cases. Concern about rumours of an epidemic can lead to improved recognition and reporting in health facilities, which result in a dramatic rise in reported cases, when there is no real increase in disease.

For certain diseases (e.g. cholera, yellow fever, viral haemorrhagic fever and plague in a non-endemic area) one confirmed case should be considered an epidemic and should prompt emergency action (see Table 2).

Assessing the impact on health

Estimating the population at risk

Review census figures or population estimates provided at provincial or district level. Determine the size and characteristics (e.g. sex and age distribution) of the population in the affected area.

Case-finding and estimating geographical distribution

The purpose of case-finding is to:

— monitor changes in the number of cases over time; and
— identify the geographical distribution of the epidemic and its possible spread to other areas.

Case-finding should include:

— interviewing health workers to detect past cases and stimulate reporting of future cases;
— reviewing outpatient, inpatient, laboratory and death records;
— investigating contacts of confirmed and suspected cases; and
— enhancing or establishing routine surveillance for this disease.

Case-finding should be based on the working case definition. It should not be limited to hospitals and urban areas only as these may provide a non-representative picture of the outbreak. This approach may lead to an underestimate of the true distribution of cases, particularly in areas where the population has poor access to health facilities. Rapid household surveys in the affected area(s) may lead to a more accurate appreciation of the epidemic.

Collecting information on all or a representative sample of cases

Careful interviewing and physical examination of identified cases is extremely important. These early clinical findings provide clues to the type of infection, source of infection, and mode of transmission.

As a minimum, gather information on:

— name, age, sex, place of residence, date of onset and date of reporting;
— signs and symptoms, severity of illness, outcome, treatment given and response to treatment; and
— presence of risk factors in order to draw conclusions about possible mode(s) of transmission.

Analysing the information

The information should be analysed in terms of time, place, and person.

Time: When did cases occur? Is the number increasing?

• Draw a simple graph showing the number of cases reported per unit of time for the course of the epidemic so far (epidemic curve).
• If the epidemic has affected a wide area, draw graphs for the different communities affected, showing the number of cases reported per unit of time.

Place: Where have cases occurred? Is the outbreak spreading? Are there accessible health facilities in affected areas?

• Map the cases geographically, if possible, by date of onset.
• Calculate the area-specific attack rate to identify areas at highest risk.
• Use maps that have settlements and health facilities indicated. If these are not available, sketch a rough map, including this information.

Person: Which groups are at greatest risk?

• Calculate specific attack rates to identify highest risk groups.
• Calculate attack rates for risk factors to identify modes of transmission.
• Estimate the numbers of hospital admissions and outpatient attendances by affected areas and by specific facilities.

These initial conclusions are necessary to guide immediate control measures and further field investigations. For instance, if the cause of the outbreak and mode(s) of transmission can be identified at this early stage, immediate action can be taken to contain the spread of the disease.

Assessing the local response capacity and immediate needs

Local response capacity

• Can local epidemic surveillance be guaranteed with existing personnel, transport, and communications?
• Are diagnostic capabilities of local laboratory and clinical services adequate?
• Are local resources sufficient for carrying out more extensive field investigations?

- Do local health facilities have sufficient staff? Are they equipped to manage adequately existing or anticipated patient load? Are they equipped to isolate patients and protect health workers?
- What steps have local health officials taken to organize epidemic response? Is there a plan of action, standardized reporting procedures, and trained staff? What steps have been taken to interrupt transmission?
- What links have been established with key community members (e.g. for education, improved case detection, and protection of uncontaminated water sources)?
- What are the existing stocks and supplies of key drugs, vaccines, and laboratory reagents?

Immediate needs

Look for needs in the following areas:

— epidemiological expertise to maintain adequate surveillance and carry out further investigation;
— laboratory support (e.g. shipment of specimens to national and international reference laboratories or imports of necessary equipment);
— environmental control (e.g. improving water quality);
— qualified clinical personnel and training for case management;
— isolation of patients and protection of health workers;
— essential medicines, vaccines and equipment; and
— transportation, communication and logistics.

Presenting results

In presenting the results of your assessment, indicate the following:

- Estimate geographical magnitude and health impact in numbers of projected cases and deaths.
- Estimate needs for outside assistance based on preliminary findings (e.g. drugs, vaccines, technical personnel, and logistics and communications support).
- Give recommendations on the following:
  — priority activities and priority at-risk groups, if the disease has been diagnosed; refer to existing emergency plans that may have been prepared; and
  — further epidemiological field investigations, if the epidemic is still not well understood.
- Convey the rapid assessment findings to decision-makers at community, subnational, national and international levels.

Chapter 3

Meningitis outbreaks

Purpose of assessment

The purpose of this rapid assessment is to:

— confirm that an epidemic or potential epidemic of meningococcal meningitis exists and estimate its geographical distribution;
— estimate its health impact; and
— assess local response capacity and identify the most effective control measures to minimize the outbreak's ill effects.

Background

Geographical distribution

Meningococcal meningitis, caused by the organism *Neisseria meningitidis*, is responsible for epidemic emergencies that are particularly severe in sub-Saharan Africa. In areas within the "meningitis belt", epidemics occur in 8 to 12 year cycles and are characterized by attack rates as high as 1%, mortality rates of up to 10%, even with treatment, and neurological sequelae among survivors.

However, outbreaks of meningococcal disease have reached other African countries. The epidemics seen towards the end of the 1980s and the early 1990s in Burundi, the Central African Republic, Kenya, Rwanda, Uganda, the United Republic of Tanzania and Zambia are examples of the disease's spread outside its usual boundaries. This reflected the extension of drought areas, or increased population movements owing to voluntary travel, warfare or movements of refugees. The outbreaks may also reflect the introduction of a new meningococcal strain into susceptible populations.

Cluster outbreaks in the Eastern Mediterranean Region have also occurred through transmission at international gatherings, such as pilgrimages. At a country level, epidemics have been reported in at-risk settings such as refugee camps, military facilities, and disadvantaged communities. The risk of person-to-person transmission is greatly increased in these populations since the disease is spread through respiratory droplets from cases with nasopharyngitis or from asymptomatic carriers.

Recently, Mongolia has experienced epidemics of magnitude comparable to that of the meningitis belt. India and Nepal also had serious outbreaks in the mid-1990s.

Epidemic threshold

For countries with high rates of endemic meningitis, such as those within the traditional meningitis belt, a rate of 15 cases per 100000 per week in a given area, averaged over two consecutive weeks, appears to be a sensitive and specific predictor of epidemic disease in this area.

In areas where epidemic meningococcal disease is unusual, a three- to four-fold increase in cases compared with a similar time period in previous years may indicate an epidemic. Another potentially useful indicator of an emerging epidemic in areas outside the meningitis belt is a doubling of meningitis cases from one week to the next for a period of three weeks. This criterion may be used, for example, in countries where population data are not available, in refugee camps, and in closed communities.

Vaccines

Vaccines are currently available to prevent meningococcal meningitis caused by serogroups A, C, Y and W135, usually provided as bivalent A and C, or quadrivalent vaccines.

A single dose of group A vaccine protects those over one to two years of age. Data show that antibody levels rise within 7 to 10 days of vaccination. Children of three months to two years of age may benefit from a second dose, although the vaccine's efficacy has not been proven for this age group. The duration of protection in adults is at least three years.

Group C vaccine has not been shown to be effective in children under two years old.

Treatment

A single intramuscular injection of long-acting chloramphenicol in oil has been proved effective in meningococcal meningitis epidemics. If there is no clinical improvement after 24 to 48 hours, a second dose should be given. Penicillin, ampicillin, and chloramphenicol are also effective, but require multiple doses and, in severe cases, intravenous administration.

Conducting the assessment

Although a functioning health surveillance system should detect any unusual increase in the number of meningitis cases, meningitis epidemics are often first reported by hospitals, community leaders or the media.

In any instance, a rapid assessment is necessary.

It is important to choose a sufficiently large population for the assessment of weekly attack rates, at least 30 000 to 50 000 since disease rates in smaller populations can fluctuate widely even with a small number of cases. On the other hand, if only very large (>1 000 000) populations are observed, low overall attack rates may obscure high rates within smaller populations in local areas. The most appropriate denominators are administrative areas with population ranging between 30 000 and 100 000.

The decision to call for an emergency response to a meningococcal meningitis outbreak is determined by:

— the seriousness of its health impact on the population at risk; and
— the ability of local health services to respond.

These two factors should be given priority during the assessment.

The rapid assessment consists of confirming a meningitis outbreak and estimating its geographical distribution, assessing the health impact, and the local response capacity and immediate needs.

Confirming a meningitis outbreak and estimating its geographical distribution

To confirm the existence of a meningitis outbreak and estimate its geographical distribution, establish an initial case definition, undertake case-findings, and collect appropriate specimens for laboratory analysis and confirmation.

Initial case definition

The initial case definition is best determined in advance, as part of emergency preparedness. Simple, viable case definitions should be determined for infants, older children, and adults.

The standard case definition of bacterial meningitis[1] is as follows:

- *Suspected case.*[2] Sudden onset of elevated temperature (>38.5 °C rectal or 38.0 °C axillary) with stiff neck or petechial or purpural rash or both.

  In patients under one year of age, a suspected case of meningitis occurs when fever is accompanied by a bulging fontanelle.

- *Probable case.*[3] Suspected case as defined above with turbid cerebrospinal fluid (CSF) (with or without positive Gram stain) or ongoing epidemic.
- *Confirmed case.*[4] Suspected or probable case as defined above and either positive cerebrospinal fluid (CSF) antigen detection or positive culture.

Case-finding

Case-finding is best undertaken through hospitals and other health facilities in the affected area. A rapid survey of households is probably not useful as, even in serious epidemics, the attack rate may not exceed 5 per 1000.

By reviewing hospital records for the same period during previous years, it may be possible to determine whether there is a significant increase in cases. Look at their geographical distribution, and at the speed at which new cases are being reported.

---

[1] This case definition allows the detection of meningococcal septicaemia.
[2] Often the only diagnosis that can be made in dispensaries (peripheral level of health care).
[3] Diagnosed in health centres where lumbar puncture and CSF examination are feasible (intermediate level).
[4] Diagnosed in well-equipped hospitals (provincial or central level).

Collection of specimens

In areas where meningitis is hyperendemic or periodically epidemic, clinical recognition is usually reliable. However, every effort should be made to obtain CSF from cases. This is essential to:

— confirm the diagnosis and define the serogroup to determine whether vaccination is a useful strategy; and
— determine antimicrobial sensitivity for treatment and possible prophylaxis.

If routine bacteriological capability is available, CSF specimens can be plated and incubated on site (e.g. in an equipped provincial hospital).

Although diagnosis in the field can be undertaken by examining a smear of CSF, the results may be unreliable. In such cases, CSF specimens should be transported under sterile conditions for analysis at a laboratory equipped with commercially available antigen detection kits.

The following considerations are important in specimen collection:

• While it is preferable to obtain CSF specimens before antibiotic therapy has begun, treatment should not be delayed. Rather, it should be noted on the form accompanying the specimen that antibiotics have already been administered.
• If adequate laboratory capacity is not available, CSF specimens can be inoculated into transport-isolation media on site, and then transported to an equipped laboratory (screw-top tubes are less likely to become contaminated in field conditions than plates).
• If transport media are not available, then CSF should be collected in a clean and sterile container for transport to a suitably equipped laboratory.

To verify the laboratory diagnosis and confirm the organism serogroup and antibiotic sensitivities, it is advisable to ship specimens to WHO collaborating centres for urgent analysis.

Assessing the impact on health

To assess the impact on health of a meningitis outbreak, collect information on sample cases, analyse the information gathered, and draw initial conclusions.

Collecting information on a sample of cases

Time and resources permitting, information on age, sex, occupation, residence, and date of onset is helpful in identifying groups at greatest risk from:

— the spread of the disease (e.g. overcrowded squatter settlements where the potential risk of rapid transmission is great); and
— mortality (e.g. identify populations with poor access to health facilities and those with poorly equipped health facilities where a higher mortality risk might be expected).

Analysing the information

Time: When did cases occur? Is the number increasing?

- Draw a simple graph to show the number of cases reported per day for the epidemic so far.
- If the meningitis outbreak has affected a wide area, construct simple graphs for the different areas affected.

Place: Where have meningitis cases occurred? Is the outbreak spreading? Are there accessible health facilities in affected areas?

- Map cases geographically if possible by date of onset.
- Use maps that identify settlements, health facilities, and major transport routes. If these are not available, sketch a rough map including this information. This helps identify at-risk areas and their relation to road or rail links and existing health facilities that are important for organizing a rapid response.

Person: Which groups and communities are at greatest risk? How many cases are there so far, or could there be in the future?

- Estimate the number of hospital admissions and clinic attendances for affected areas and for specific facilities.

Drawing initial conclusions on the outbreak
To draw initial conclusions about the outbreak, you should obtain answers to the following questions:

- Is there an outbreak of acute meningococcal meningitis?
- How many cases and deaths so far?
- What is the geographical distribution of the cases?
- What is the size of the population at risk?
- Is the outbreak spreading? Where?
- What do preliminary laboratory results show?

Assessing local response capacity and immediate needs
Local response capacity and immediate needs should be assessed to determine the type and quantity of external support required.

Local epidemiological surveillance
- Are more extensive field investigations needed?
- If the outbreak has affected a large population or has occurred in an area inaccessible to the capital or both, is there at least one available person with training in epidemiology to maintain and supervise outbreak surveillance?
- Will she or he have available an appropriate vehicle to visit the area affected?
- Is outside help needed?

Response capacity of local health services
- What is the case-fatality ratio?
- What steps have local health officials taken to organize epidemic response? Is there a plan of action, standardized reporting procedures, and trained staff?

- What linkages have been established with key community leaders (e.g. to improve case detection and allay panic)?
- Are health facilities accessible to affected populations? Are temporary centres needed? Where?
- Is there at least one qualified physician in the affected area experienced in the clinical management of meningitis?
- At district-level facilities, is there at least one nurse or health worker with experience in the care of severely ill meningitis patients?
- Are health facilities equipped and do they have sufficient staff for projected patient load?
- What is the local cold chain capacity? Are there trained vaccinators, jet injectors, vehicles, stocks of syringes and vaccines?
- Is there access to vehicles for local distribution and supply of emergency drugs?
- What stocks of drugs (e.g. oily and oral chloramphenicol, crystalline benzylpenicillin, and supportive drugs) are available?

Determine immediate needs

When deciding on the need for emergency response the following questions should be considered.

- Is there an outbreak of meningococcal meningitis that has or could lead to a large number of cases?
- If so, are outside resources needed to contain it?

If the answer to both questions is "yes", then an emergency response is needed.

Presenting results

When presenting the results of the rapid health assessment indicate the following:

 — confirm the serogroup responsible for the outbreak and determine antibiotic sensitivities as urgent priorities, if still unknown;
 — describe the situation; and
 — recommend action.

Describe the situation

- Give an estimate of the geographical magnitude and potential health impact by determining the size of the population at risk and the number of projected cases, hospital admissions, and deaths.
- Quantify the available resources and the need for outside assistance based on these preliminary findings (e.g. vaccines, drugs, and logistics and communications support).

Recommend action

- If the epidemic is caused by serogroups A or C, immediate immunization should begin.
- If sufficient vaccine supplies and administrative support are available, mass vaccination of the entire population should be considered.

- If resources are limited, it may be necessary to restrict vaccination to the age groups most at risk, namely those with the highest attack rates or accounting for the largest proportion of cases.
- Prepare and convey assessment findings to epidemic emergency decision-makers at community, subnational, national, and international levels.

Chapter 4

Outbreaks of viral haemorrhagic fever, including yellow fever

Purpose of assessment

The purpose of this rapid assessment is to:

— confirm that an epidemic or potential epidemic of viral haemorrhagic fever (VHF) exists and estimate its geographical distribution;
— estimate its health impact; and
— assess local response capacity and identify the most effective control measures.

Background

General characteristics

Viral haemorrhagic fevers (VHF) are caused by a number of viruses, some associated with insects or rodents, which may infect humans. These diseases cause special problems for public health services because of their epidemic potential, high case-fatality rates and the unusual difficulties arising in their treatment and prevention.

While the specific clinical profile of each viral illness may vary, there are two prominent symptoms that may appear in all types of VHF during the most critical stage of the illness:

— bleeding, with the risk of severe haemorrhage from both cutaneous and internal sites; and
— the development of shock, which may be irreversible.

The existence of a specific virus in a community tends to reflect the geographical distribution of its natural host. Nevertheless, human and natural environments are changing rapidly so research should be considered an integral part of emergency preparedness against these epidemics.

Several viral infections also have the potential for extensive nosocomial spread (spread within a health care facility), especially when safe barrier nursing procedures are not observed. Under these conditions, case-fatality rates can often exceed 50% and may reach 80% for several days.

Table 3 lists the major VHFs that cause epidemics and shows their distribution.

Table 3. **Viral haemorrhagic fevers causing epidemics**

VHF	Distribution	Natural host/vector
Lassa fever	Central/West Africa	rodents
Junin/Machupo/Guanarito/Sabia	South America	rodents
Ebola/Marburg	Africa	unknown
Crimean-Congo haemorrhagic fever (CCHF)	Africa/Asia	ticks
Rift Valley fever	Africa	mosquitos
Dengue haemorrhagic fever	Africa/Americas/Pacific/ western Asia/ Australasia/Caribbean/ India	mosquitos
Yellow fever	Africa/South America	mosquitos
Haemorrhagic fever with renal syndrome (HFRS)	Asia/Europe	rodents

The special concerns of yellow fever

In Africa and South America, yellow fever has caused many serious epidemics, with high attack rates and mortality. However, while the clinical presentation of yellow fever may resemble other types of VHF, it is unique with respect to emergency preparedness and containment. Unlike other VHFs, timely vaccination against yellow fever, combined with vector control measures, interrupts transmission and prevents unnecessary cases and deaths.

There are many examples of yellow fever epidemics that were identified as such several months after the actual epidemic onset. The consequences of this late detection (e.g. delayed initiation of control efforts) underscore the need to consider yellow fever in a rapid assessment when an outbreak of VHF is reported or rumoured.

An epidemic alert for an outbreak of VHF with yellow fever as a possible cause should be given when one of the following occurs:

- one case is confirmed in a community with abundant vector mosquitos;
- a single case of yellow fever is diagnosed by serology or virus isolation, or suggested by histopathology;
- hospital reports show increased incidence of fatal hepatitis, suspected cases of yellow fever and of VHF.

Early warning procedures such as routine health surveillance and rapid reporting from hospitals are essential for detecting VHF outbreaks at an early stage.

The questions below should be addressed as part of these early warning procedures:

- Where are the high-risk areas for past and potential VHF and yellow fever epidemics? At-risk populations? Based on past experience, when are the high-risk seasons?
- What is the likely health impact of an epidemic of VHF or yellow fever (number of cases, hospitalizations, and deaths)?
- What early signs would signal a VHF or yellow fever "epidemic alert"? Can or could they be detected earlier through improved epidemic surveillance and reporting?
- Does routine health surveillance include rural areas, where VHF outbreaks frequently occur?

When VHF outbreaks are reported, they receive heavy media coverage, often in the context of the panic such outbreaks arouse in the local medical services and communities affected. Rapid health assessments will provide factual evidence on the existence and extent of an outbreak. This information can be provided to the media so that the potentially affected population and the medical authorities can make informed decisions.

In this way, the rapid assessment offers a valuable opportunity to allay the community's anxiety and to provide basic information on protective measures to prevent the disease's further spread.

Preparedness

Develop locally adapted working case definitions for VHFs and yellow fever, as well as guidelines to help health workers at all levels recognize suspicious trends and signal an epidemic alert.

The prompt diagnosis of a VHF outbreak's cause requires a competent laboratory's analysis of a representative sample of specimens. Epidemic preparedness should give this utmost priority, along with assessing the capacity of national laboratories; identifying reference laboratories; and ensuring methods of diagnostic specimen transport.

Most of the viruses causing VHF (excluding dengue haemorrhagic fever) are classified as "Biosafety Level 4" pathogens. This biohazard requires analysis at special facilities that provide maximum containment.

Attempts to isolate the virus should be undertaken only at approved high containment laboratories. Therefore, these should be identified in advance and contacts established with the nearest specialist laboratory to obtain details of necessary precautions for packing and transport of specimens.

Serology can be carried out in standard laboratories only if it is possible to inactivate specimens and reagents.

The measures listed below should also be taken:

- identify in advance qualified local team members skilled in assessing VHF outbreaks (e.g. an epidemiologist, clinician/entomologist, virologist, and veterinarian);

— put in place advance provisions for obtaining rapid outside specialist support if qualified personnel are not locally available;
— obtain advice from a virologist on the specimens needed, precautions required for collection, the necessary equipment, and shipment procedures (consider International Air Transport Association (IATA) shipping restrictions);
— identify channels and means for rapid communication between peripheral areas and subnational/central levels — satellite telephone and facsimile may be required; and
— identify a knowledgeable individual to communicate with the press and develop a strategy to deal effectively with their inquiries.

Conducting the assessment

The rapid assessment consists of confirming an outbreak of VHF and estimating its geographical distribution, assessing the impact on health, and determining the existing response capacity and immediate needs.

Confirming an outbreak of VHF and estimating its geographical distribution

Initial case definition
As for all potential epidemics, this is best determined in advance, as part of emergency preparedness. Simple, viable case definitions should be developed for suspect, probable, and confirmed cases of VHF.

Examples of case definitions for VHF are:

• *Suspected case:* acute fever with either jaundice, or cutaneous and internal bleeding, accompanied by shock; in the case of dengue the rash should also be mentioned.
• *Probable case:* a suspected case with at least two of the following signs: severe myalgia and headache, conjunctivitis, rash, shock, proteinuria, death, where the person has had contact with a possible source of transmission.
• *Confirmed case:* a suspected or probable case with one of the following: virus isolation from blood or tissue; detection of viral antigen or genome in blood, tissue or other body fluid; presence of specific IgM antibody in titre high enough to indicate recent infection.

In a rapid assessment, it may be difficult to distinguish yellow fever from other haemorrhagic illnesses or diseases such as malaria. However, to maximize case detection at this early stage, it is often necessary to use a broad case definition such as "jaundice, fatal or non-fatal" to identify suspected cases.

Confirming the increase in the number of cases
(See Chapter 2, p. 20.)

Case-finding and estimating geographical distribution
(See Chapter 2, p. 20.)

It is important to recognize that there could be many asymptomatic or mild cases who are hospitalized with a non-specific febrile illness. To be thorough, VHF and yellow fever case-finding efforts should not be limited to infectious wards but include other hospital departments and health facilities.

Collection of specimens

Because the definitive diagnosis of a VHF can only be made by serology or virus isolation, it is essential that appropriate specimens be collected during the rapid assessment.

Key considerations in specimen collection are as follows:

- Essential information should be included with specimens (locality, name of patient, age, sex, date of sampling, date of disease onset, and summary of clinical and epidemiological findings).
- All specimens should be collected in sterile containers.
- All specimens must be considered potentially infectious and dangerous. Therefore, stringent safety precautions should be observed.
- For every patient, a specimen of whole blood should be collected without anticoagulant for virus isolation or antibody detection.
- Do not freeze whole blood or liver specimens: separate sera if specimens are to be frozen.
- All sera and cerebrospinal fluid (CSF) specimens should be frozen for preservation during transport. For virus isolation, specifically, specimens should be stored ideally on liquid nitrogen or dry ice.
- Specimens are best hand-carried from peripheral areas to the central level.
- Use non-breakable containers (plastic, screw-cap) with absorbent material to contain any leakage, and double outer containers. Follow International Air Transport Association (IATA) regulations for air transport of specimens.

The specimens required for laboratory analysis and confirmation are as follows:

— whole blood from patients who have been sick less than seven days (do not separate sera from blood clots unless laboratory workers can be protected against infectious aerosols);
— convalescent sera from patients at least 14 days after onset (sera should be carefully separated from blood clots);
— for suspect yellow fever cases, liver specimens should be taken at postmortem with a biopsy needle (these should be divided in two — one placed in 10% buffered formalin and the other treated in the same way as a whole blood specimen — not frozen without anticoagulant);
— skin snips preserved in formalin from fatal cases of suspect VHF.

To verify the clinical diagnosis and identify the causative virus, it is advisable to transport specimens to WHO collaborating centres for urgent analysis.

Assessing the impact on health

Collecting information on a representative sample of cases

When the cause of a VHF outbreak is unknown, careful interviewing and physical examination of suspect, probable, and confirmed cases is extremely important.

These early clinical findings provide clues as to the type of virus and source of infection.

As a minimum, gather information on:

— name, age, sex, residence, date of onset, and of reporting;
— signs and symptoms, severity of illness, treatment given, and response to treatment; and
— presence of risk factors, e.g. history of contact.

Useful information on the mode of transmission can be gained by investigating the contacts of identified index cases. It is also important to ask about exposures to infected animal hosts (e.g. contact while slaughtering livestock).

The definition of a "primary" or "close" contact is one or more of the following:

— has shared the same place (for working or travelling), the same room or meals, had occasional face-to-face contact during the period of communicability of a severe, classical or mild form of the disease;
— has given care, handled the patient's belongings, participated in autopsy or burial preparations without special protection; or
— has travelled from an area where VHF transmission is endemic.

The definition of a "possible" contact is:

— was a close contact of a case during a period in which she or he possibly was not yet contagious (e.g. persons hospitalized in the same ward).

Whatever the method chosen, the characterization of the contact should include a clarification on the index case: was he or she suspect, probable or confirmed?

Analysing the information
The information should be analysed in terms of time, place, and person (See Chapter 2).

Assess vectors present
One rapid assessment priority is to determine whether vectors that may transmit VHF or yellow fever are present in the affected area. It is not the purpose of a rapid assessment to carry out a detailed entomological survey, but rather to ask the following questions.

• Are vectors present in the affected area? If so, what are they?
• Are they known to bite humans?
• Are there breeding sites? If so, how extensive?

The answers to these preliminary questions are critical to deciding on the need for further entomological studies and control measures for vectors and natural hosts.

Assess disease in other vertebrate hosts
• Are there unexplained deaths in monkeys in the affected area? If so, where and when did they occur?

- Are there unexplained deaths or abortions in livestock? If so, where and when did they occur? (Particularly relevant for Rift Valley fever.)

Assessing local response capacity and immediate needs

Local response capacity and immediate needs should be assessed to determine the type and quantity of external support required.

Local epidemic surveillance

- Are there sufficient trained personnel, vehicles, and communications support to maintain adequate surveillance? Is outside technical help needed?
- Is there a need for animal studies (e.g. sentinel herd surveillance) or further entomological investigations?

Response capacity of local health services

- What steps have local health officials taken to organize epidemic response? Is there a plan of action, standardized reporting procedures, and trained staff?
- Are hospitals equipped to carry out safe barrier nursing measures? (Check bed nets, gloves, disinfectants, masks, and gowns.)
- What is the local cold chain capacity? Trained vaccinators? Jet injectors? Vehicles? Stocks of syringes? Yellow fever vaccine stocks in country?
- Do medical, nursing and laboratory personnel need further training on case detection and safe patient management?
- What links have been established with key community members (e.g. for allaying panic in case of outbreaks, for general health education and improved surveillance and case detection)?
- What vector control equipment, pesticides, and larvicides are available?
- Has a strategy been developed for dealing with press inquiries?

Determine immediate needs

To determine immediate needs the following questions should be addressed.

- Is there an outbreak of VHF which has led or could lead to a large number of cases?
- If so, are external resources needed to contain it?

If the answer to both questions is "yes", then an emergency response is needed.

Presenting results

In presenting the results of your assessment, indicate the following information:

- Is there an outbreak of some type of VHF?
- If so, how many cases and deaths so far?
- What is the geographical distribution?
- Does it appear to be spreading?
- What are the trends?
- What is the clinical presentation?
- Are signs and symptoms indicative of any specific type of VHF?
- Where should specimens be sent for rapid analysis?
- Is the etiologic agent responsible for the outbreak identified?

- Have specimens been sent to reference laboratories?
- What are the estimated geographical magnitude, size of population at risk and health impact in numbers of projected cases and deaths?

Describe the immediate needs. Are outside resources (such as drugs, equipment, other supplies, personnel, expert assistance, logistics, funding) needed?

Chapter 5

Outbreaks of acute diarrhoeal disease

Purpose of assessment

The purpose of this rapid health assessment is to:

— confirm that an epidemic of acute diarrhoeal disease exists and estimate its geographical distribution;
— estimate its health impact; and
— assess existing response capacity and identify the most effective control measures to minimize the outbreak's ill effects.

Background

In many places, diarrhoeal diseases are endemic with seasonal peaks. However, when serious outbreaks of acute diarrhoeal disease occur, the common cause is either:

— *Shigella dysenteriae* type 1 (Sd1), which causes bacillary dysentery, or
— *Vibrio cholerae* serogroup O1 or O139, which causes cholera.

Shigella dysenteriae type 1 (Sd1)

This is the most virulent of the four serogroups of shigellae, and is often resistant to most of the common antimicrobials. The illness caused by Sd1 often includes abdominal cramps, fever, and rectal pain. Less frequent complications with Sd1 include sepsis, seizures, renal failure, and haemolytic/uraemic syndrome. The organism is highly infectious, and readily transmitted by direct person-to-person contact as well as by food and water.

Shigella dysentery type 1 always should be considered as a possible cause of the outbreak when there is an unusual increase in the weekly number of cases of bloody diarrhoea or deaths from bloody diarrhoea.

Vibrio cholerae O1 and O139

Cholera has spread widely since 1961 and now affects at least 98 countries.

Most people infected have no symptoms or only mild diarrhoea. However, those with a severe case of the disease can die within hours of onset from fluid/electrolyte loss through profuse diarrhoea and, to a lesser extent, vomiting. Although high death rates can occur when treatment is unavailable, case fatality can be reduced to below 1% with proper facilities and care. The organism is spread almost exclusively by ingestion of food or water contaminated directly or indirectly by faeces or vomit from infected individuals.

A cholera outbreak should be suspected if either or both of the following occur:

— a patient older than five years develops severe dehydration or dies from acute watery diarrhoea;
— there is a sudden increase in the daily number of patients with acute watery diarrhoea, especially patients who pass the "rice water" stools typical of cholera.

Conducting the assessment

The rapid assessment consists of confirming an outbreak of acute diarrhoeal disease, assessing the impact on health, the existing response capacity, and additional immediate needs.

The assessment team should be equipped with specimen containers and sufficient transport media (such as Cary-Blair) for collecting specimens to analyse at the closest competent laboratory.

Confirming an outbreak of acute diarrhoeal disease

Confirming the clinical diagnosis and collection of specimens
This can be carried out by examining a number of cases. Confirming the outbreak and implementing control measures should not await laboratory results. However, for both dysentery and cholera, reliable laboratory techniques are essential for confirming the clinical diagnosis and determining antimicrobial sensitivities.

Initial case definition
As in all rapid epidemic assessments, this is an important first step for guiding early field investigations and identifying cases. Standard case definitions for suspected cases of acute diarrhoeal disease are:

- In an area where the disease is not known to be present, a patient aged five years or more develops severe dehydration or dies from acute watery diarrhoea.
- In an area where there is a cholera epidemic, a patient aged five years or more develops acute watery diarrhoea, with or without vomiting.[1]
- A case of cholera is confirmed when *Vibrio cholerae* O1 or O139 is isolated from any patient with diarrhoea.
- Bacillary dysentery is confirmed by evidence of acute onset of bloody diarrhoea with visible blood in the stool.

[1] For management of cases of acute watery diarrhoea in an area where there is a cholera epidemic, cholera should be suspected in all patients aged two years or more. However, the inclusion of all cases of acute watery diarrhoea in the two- to four-year age group in the reporting of cholera greatly reduces the specificity of reporting.

Assessing the impact on health

Case-finding and estimating geographical distribution

In endemic areas, cases of cholera and bacillary dysentery occur every year, usually with seasonal peaks. Therefore, it is extremely important for the rapid assessment to determine whether there are significantly more cases than should be expected.

Active case-finding is needed to determine the size of the outbreak, based on the initial case definitions. Cholera and bacillary dysentery can be distinguished by their clinical presentations (see p. 38).

Collecting information on a representative sample of cases

Focus on what is already known about patterns of spread for both bacillary dysentery and cholera to identify possible sources of the outbreak and means of spread. The case-fatality ratio should be calculated and used to assess the adequacy of patient management.

The case-fatality ratio should be <1% for cholera, and from 1% to 10% during epidemics of Sd1.

- *Cholera:* Because spread can occur by contaminated food and water, or more rarely by person-to-person contact in overcrowded conditions, ask questions about possible types of exposure.
- *Bacillary dysentery:* Because spread can occur through contaminated food or water or direct person-to-person transmission, ask questions to determine how spread is occurring.

Analysing the information

Time: When did the cases occur? Is their number increasing? Did many people become ill at the same time at the outbreak's beginning?

- Draw a simple graph to show the number of cases reported per day so far.
- If the diarrhoeal disease outbreak has affected a wide area, construct simple graphs for the different areas affected, showing the number of cases reported per day.

Place: Where have cases occurred? Is the outbreak spreading? How is it spreading?

- Map cases geographically, by date of onset.

Use maps that identify water sources, settlements, health facilities and major transport routes. If they are not available, sketch a rough map including this information. This helps to identify at-risk areas and their relation to road and rail links and existing health facilities, which are important for organizing a rapid response.

Person: Which groups are at greatest risk (e.g. age, occupations)? How many cases are there so far, or could there be in the future?

- Calculate overall attack rates.
- Calculate age-specific and sex-specific attack rates.
- Estimate the number of cases in the future.

In past epidemics, attack rates for clinical cholera have been about 0.2%. However, in a severe epidemic the attack rate has been as high as 1%. In order to calculate supply needs for the first weeks, a bacillary dysentery attack rate of 2% can be assumed. Information on the treatment of cholera and dysentery is contained in Box 1.

Assessing local response capacity and immediate needs
The following questions are guidelines for assessing the local response capacity and determining the need for outside resources.

Response capacity of local health services
- What steps have local health officials taken to organize the epidemic response? Is there a plan of action, standardized reporting procedures, and trained staff?
- Are guidelines for management prepared and followed? What is the case-fatality ratio?
- Are all supplies for treatment readily available (oral rehydration salts (ORS), antibiotics, intravenous (IV) fluids, soap, and chlorine)?
- What links have been established with key community leaders (e.g. to facilitate health education, improve case detection, and protect water sources)?
- Are health facilities accessible to the affected populations? Are temporary treatment centres needed?
- Are there sufficient trained health workers to treat cases properly?
- Are resources being diverted to ineffective control measures, such as trade or travel restrictions?

Local epidemiological surveillance
- Are there sufficient trained personnel, vehicles, laboratory and communications support to maintain surveillance? Is outside help needed?
- Are more extensive field investigations needed?
- Can surveillance of diarrhoea cases and environmental sources (particularly sewage, using Moore swabs) be maintained until *Vibrio cholerae* O1 or O139 is no longer isolated from people and the environment in non-endemic areas?

Presenting results

In presenting the results of the assessment, indicate the following information.

- Whether there is an outbreak of acute diarrhoeal disease.
- If the clinical diagnosis is confirmed by laboratory tests.
- The number of cases and deaths so far.
- The geographical distribution of the cases.

- The size of the population at risk.
- If the outbreak is spreading and where.
- Whether antimicrobial sensitivities have been assessed.
- Whether emergency plans for epidemic control have been implemented.
- Whether national and international reporting is occurring.
- How satisfactory the case management is.

Box 1. **Treatment of cholera and dysentery**

Cholera
The mainstay of treatment is ORS or — in severe cases — intravenous fluids until oral fluids can be taken. Antimicrobial treatment will shorten the duration of illness, decrease excretion of vibrios and reduce fluid loss — but is not essential for successful treatment and should be reserved for severe cases only.

Epidemic dysentery (Sd1)
Selection of appropriate antimicrobials should be based on laboratory results of resistance patterns.

Chapter 6

Sudden-impact natural disasters

Purpose of assessment

A rapid assessment should be initiated as soon as possible after a natural disaster to determine:

— the type of emergency, the affected areas and population, and the emergency's likely evolution;
— its impact on health;
— the immediate impact on health services; and
— the extent of damage to other sectors relevant to health operations.

Background

In addition to killing and injuring people and causing extensive environmental, social, and economic damage, sudden-impact natural disasters often create an immediate obstacle to response by disrupting vital services (e.g. water, health, and security services) as well as key communication and transportation systems.

Sudden-impact natural disasters can be triggered by:

— cyclones, hurricanes, tornadoes;
— snowstorms;
— tsunamis (seismically induced waves);
— storm surges;
— flash floods;
— fires;
— earthquakes;
— landslides and avalanches; and
— volcanic eruptions.

The impact of any one of these hazards upon a vulnerable population can cause a disaster. Nonetheless, natural hazards occur in well-defined patterns. Susceptible areas can be rather easily identified, and therefore emergency plans should be prepared that outline administrative and technical responsibilities and procedures for a health response to all likely natural disasters. These plans should be multisectoral and linked to any other existing emergency plans.

Priorities

Disasters, emergencies, and the required response can be viewed in terms of stages, and the type of information collected must be appropriate for every stage of the emergency response.

Stage I (Day 1)

The first response in sudden-impact disasters comes from the affected community, and local priorities are to simultaneously assess and respond rapidly to the crisis. This implies that medical measures are usually implemented without complete information. Local resources are spontaneously and, often, effectively reassigned and adjusted before the first results of a rapid assessment are available.

During this period, when additional resources have not yet arrived, the highest health priority is the emergency medical response.

The first injury estimates are needed within the 24 hours following impact to guide requests for assistance. However, in many sudden-impact disasters, it is difficult to project numbers of casualties during this period. An important task of preparedness is to review the experience gained in past disasters (e.g. earthquakes and floods) and prepare guidelines for estimating casualties (for instance, in the case of earthquakes, based on recorded magnitude, population density, and construction type).

Stage II (Day 2)

By this time, most critical patients in accessible areas have already received initial medical attention and immediate life-saving measures become less important.

During this stage, a rapid assessment should determine:

— needs for emergency medical response in the less accessible areas;
— shortages in primary health care resources;
— secondary needs: health care, shelter, food and water for the population; and
— needs for additional national and international resources (to re-establish essential health services, and restock medical supplies and equipment).

Stage III (Days 3–5)

At this point, restoring primary health care, lifeline systems, and adequate shelter become priorities.

Therefore, a rapid assessment should focus progressively on needs for:

— environmental health, food security and safety, and public health services;
— special protection and shelter for vulnerable groups; and
— re-establishing the primary health care system, and restoring health facilities.

Stage IV (after Day 5)

After day 5, emergency plans should be fully implemented, and a response and recovery operation ideally in place, covering all sectors.

From this stage on, health assessment should:

— be based on an established surveillance system;
— incorporate information on both disease surveillance, and the health care system;
— focus on health trends as they relate to the response and recovery operation itself; and
— contribute to the most effective use of national and international resources.

Conducting the assessment

The information collected must highlight the population and areas most severely affected, the damage to the health system, and the status of affected and unaffected health resources. Information previously obtained from other sources (such as government departments) should be included in the assessment. Rapid assessment activities should provide the basis for establishing ongoing surveillance.

Estimating the disaster's impact on a population requires basic demographic information (such as age and sex distribution of the population) and a good knowledge of the affected area (for example, the mapped location of health facilities, water sources, and high-risk communities). This information is often available from government departments, academic institutions or response and recovery organizations.

Assessing the impact on health

Injuries
Primary injuries: Injury patterns and their importance vary according to the type of disaster. For example, earthquakes are associated with a large number of traumatic injuries, while floods are often associated with many deaths, but relatively few injuries. A rapid assessment should:

— estimate the number of persons injured; and
— assess the severity of injuries (using a simple scale for ranking severity, such as "those requiring and not requiring hospitalization within 24 hours").

Other useful information includes:

— types of injuries (such as laceration, fracture, and burns);
— injury sites (such as arm, back, leg, and head); and
— approximate age and sex distribution of affected persons.

Secondary injuries: Secondary injuries may occur in the post-impact phase of a disaster:

— from secondary effects of the disaster, such as fires and toxic releases; and
— in association with the clean-up and rescue operations, and as people return to their homes. Risk groups include residents, response and rescue workers, volunteers, and others in the affected area.

Methods for collecting information: Potential sources of information include any place where the injured may have gone to seek care. The number of seriously injured is more important than the number of ambulatory patients. Therefore, information should be collected from second- and third-level health facilities, where most of the seriously injured seek help (see Table 4).

Information may be obtained by site visits or contacting the officers responsible. As soon as possible, a surveillance system should be established to monitor changing health conditions.

Missing persons

Other critical information for determining the severity of a sudden-impact natural disaster is the number of persons who are missing or unaccounted for. Information on their possible location and expected health condition may be needed to plan the medical aspects of search and rescue operations.

An accurate tally of missing persons and the number of dead bodies recovered will be essential, at least at a late stage of the operations (see Deaths, p. 47).

Information sources include the following:

- Preliminary indications will come from interviews with the families of the missing persons and the community at large (e.g. through a survey).
- The most important sources for this information are those entities which are responsible for search and rescue: i.e. the police, army and fire brigade.
- In some cases, schools and hotels, for example, will have registers of pupils or guests that can help in this task.

Survivors in need

Most, if not all, the survivors in the affected area, even if not physically injured, may have been left homeless and deprived of all lifeline systems and services (see Assessing the impact on health-related sectors, p. 49, and Chapter 7).

Table 4. **Gathering information to assess the health impact of a natural disaster**

When	Where: information sources
During immediate post-impact stages	• Hospitals (those with usable emergency room and inpatient records, including mobile hospitals, are the best sources)
During later stages	• Pharmacies • Community health centres • Evacuation centres • Local officials and leaders • Nongovernmental organizations • Community organizations

Many among them may also need psychological support to overcome the stress of the disaster or the loss of relatives or friends.

Obtaining figures or estimates on their number is essential to plan immediate and medium-term response and activities.

Data can be collected from:

— local officials and leaders;
— evacuation centres;
— NGOs; and
— community organizations.

Other illness

Communicable disease outbreaks are quite rare in the days immediately following a sudden natural disaster. However, with continued lack of utilities (such as water supplies and sewage treatment), disrupted health services, and poor environmental conditions, there is an increased risk of communicable disease outbreaks.

Careful consideration should be given to identifying those communicable diseases of increased risk in the disaster-affected area because only those pathogens present in the affected area are likely to cause outbreaks.

The rapid assessment should:

— identify pathogens already present, or likely to be introduced from outside the affected area (e.g. by external health workers or displaced persons or migrants from other locations); and
— identify the best measures for disease control.

Following a disaster, mass immunization campaigns are frequently unnecessary and counterproductive because they divert resources from more essential services. However, attention should be paid to the immunization status of children against measles, pertussis, diphtheria, and polio in densely populated areas.

Deaths

Mortality information is the first to be reported by the communities affected, but there are important considerations in using it.

• For immediate decision-making purposes following a sudden-impact disaster, mortality data are not as useful as information on injury patterns.
• However, for setting future priorities in emergency preparedness and response, it is useful to determine the leading causes of mortality and associated risk factors in specific types of disasters.

Key considerations in assessing information on deaths include the following.

• In a rapid-impact disaster, it may be particularly difficult to estimate the number of unrecovered bodies: reported mortality is limited to the number of bodies recovered, thus underestimating true mortality.

- It is important to differentiate between mortality estimates based on body counts, and those which include the number of people missing.
- Sources of mortality information that may be useful in a slow-onset disaster may not be useful after a rapid-impact disaster (i.e. registration of dead persons may lag in the latter case).

In addition to crude mortality information, other data can be collected after the emergency period that may be helpful in setting future preparedness priorities. They include:

— age-specific and sex-specific death rates;
— causes of death; and
— risk factors for death.

Depending on the setting and culture of the population(s) affected, the range of potential sources for mortality data includes:

— hospitals;
— cemeteries and burial grounds;
— health centres or posts;
— religious leaders;
— offices that register deaths;
— donor organizations;
— local officials and leaders; and
— NGOs.

Assessing the impact on health services

Medical services

A rapid assessment must provide essential information for determining the extent of damage, and the location of undamaged and functioning services in relation to health needs.

Immediately following the disaster or when facing time constraints, the information below should be gathered:

— number, location, and type of facilities (preferably mapped before the disaster), and previous level of functioning;
— structural integrity of health care facilities after the event;
— current capacity of health facilities;
— disrupted communications and supply lines;
— injuries and deaths of staff;
— functioning electricity and water supplies (yes or no);
— gaps in coverage by key personnel; and
— acute gaps in key supplies and medicines.

If time permits, or at a later stage, the following information may be collected:

— number and types of injuries or illnesses reported at facilities;
— needs for evacuation of injured or ill persons to other types of facilities; needs for specialized care (e.g. burn treatment);

— number and functions of medical operations (e.g. types of injuries treated and resources needed);
— number and types of medicines available, vaccines, blood, laboratory supplies, and key emergency supplies most urgently needed.

Information needed can be collected by visiting the facilities in the stricken area, or communicating by radio or telephone with outlying areas.

Environmental health

Assess the status of health-related services, such as water supply, sanitation, vector control, shelter, and transport.

Also look at secondary hazards, such as fires, chemical releases, collapse of infrastructure, such as dams, roads, and bridges that may occur after extensive structural damage in the affected area.

The priority is to assess the quantity and quality of untreated water supplies. For example, in earthquakes, ensuring an adequate quantity of water is a major problem if supply lines are cut.

Particular attention should be paid to:

— structural or functional damage to water supplies;
— size and location of populations with an adequate water supply to identify groups at increased risk of communicable disease; and
— actual or potentially contaminated water sources, and populations exposed to such sources.

In determining the state of sanitation the following should be examined:

— structural integrity of sewage treatment systems;
— signs of functional damage (such as overflowing of septic pits); and
— presence of vectors.

Floods are often associated with vector-related problems. This is due to several factors, including the emergence of new breeding sites, overcrowding in shelters and camps, and the disruption of vector control activities. Later assessment should identify the types of vectors present in the affected area, as well as the populations at increased risk of related illness.

Assessing the impact on health-related sectors

Health status and, consequently, emergency health response depend heavily on other key services. Key sectors that affect health include:

— food;
— shelter and housing; and
— transport and communication.

After a sudden-impact disaster, assessing the nutritional status is not a priority, though it is important to consider that the disaster may have affected food stocks and pipelines, and shortages may occur.

Rapid nutritional assessment will be necessary, however, if the affected population had inadequate or marginal food security before the event.

For discussion of the last two points, see Chapters 7 and 8.

Sources of error

Morbidity estimates from health care providers may not be accurate or representative.

Injuries may be under-reported owing to poor record-keeping, or because health facilities may be inaccessible for many of the injured. On the other hand, they may be over-reported because they are registered or counted several times (e.g. at the Red Cross Station, the health centre, and the hospital).

In the later stages of a sudden-impact natural disaster, other factors emerge that may reduce the usefulness of morbidity and injury data collected from health providers.

For example, the availability of health care may actually improve because of the disaster response, leading to increased medical care for both disaster-related and other injuries.

Furthermore, better diagnostic equipment in more sophisticated facilities may allow more specific or accurate diagnoses in some locations than in others. This may limit the comparability of data gathered from different sites.

A rapid assessment that concentrates on health services in the worst stricken but easily accessible areas may exaggerate the acuteness of need for the entire population affected. On the other hand, the needs of isolated areas with disrupted road, air, and telecommunications may be underestimated and easily forgotten.

Presenting results

In presenting the results of your assessment, indicate the following information.

- Describe briefly the event: site, causes and general effects, date and time of event.
- Give an estimate of the area and of the number of people affected.
- Give information on:
  — number of deaths;
  — number and pattern of injuries;
  — number of missing persons; and
  — number of people displaced or in need of being evacuated.
- Describe the extent of the damage and the current state of:
  — health facilities and services;
  — lifeline systems (water, energy, communications);
  — houses; and
  — other vital infrastructures (road, bridges, sanitation systems, etc.).

- Describe the response operations, under way or planned:
  — by the community;
  — by the local authorities;
  — by the central government;
  — by NGOs;
  — by international partners;
  — distribution of tasks and coordination mechanisms;
  — main constraints to the operations; and
  — identify other hazards that may compound the emergency.
- Give recommendations on:
  — geographical areas or population groups of priority concern;
  — activities that need to be undertaken immediately or in the short term;
  — activities that may be needed at medium term; and
  — immediate needs for external assistance such as drugs, other medical supplies, equipment, personnel, expert assistance, logistics and communications, and funding.

Chapter 7

Sudden population displacements

Purpose of assessment

The purpose of this rapid health assessment is to:

— describe the type, magnitude, and possible evolution of the displacement;
— assess the health and nutritional impact of the displacement on the displaced and host populations;
— initiate a health and nutrition surveillance system;
— assess the adequacy of existing response capacity and the immediate additional needs; and
— recommend priority actions for rapid response.

Background

People may be displaced from where they live by natural or man-made disasters, force or the threat of force, or other pressures. The term "refugee" refers to displaced persons who cross an international border. The country to which they flee is referred to as the "host country". In contrast, "internally displaced persons" do not cross an international border and remain within their country of origin.

Displaced persons may move as a large group over a short period or move in small groups over months or years. Large concentrations of displaced persons may be found in poor, peripheral, and under-served sections of large cities. The sudden arrival of large numbers (sometimes hundreds of thousands) can create a health emergency. This protocol addresses rapid health assessment in all emergencies owing to sudden displacement of both refugees and internally displaced persons.

The rapid health assessment has to include the host population because of the additional stress that may be placed on local organizations.

Conducting the assessment

The rapid assessment consists of:

— defining the area where the displaced are located;
— deciding what information to collect;
— assessing health status;

— assessing environmental conditions; and
— assessing local response capacity and additional immediate needs.

Defining the area where the displaced are located

Displaced persons may be found:

— scattered in small groups along a stretch of border, in many instances living with local villagers of the same ethnic group, or even relatives;
— massed in a relatively well-defined area near a border;
— located in transit camps organized by local officials not far from a border;
— clustered in small groups scattered along the coast of a host country, having fled by boat; and
— grouped together in urban or peri-urban settings.

Before the field assessment, review any recent information collected and compiled on the displaced group and the host areas by ministries or response and recovery organizations based in the capital city. In addition, determine whether there have been any preliminary requests, orders or actual procurement of food, medical or other emergency supplies.

Deciding what information to collect

Before the assessment, investigators must decide what information to collect, and prioritize it to ensure that the essential information will be gathered if time or resources are inadequate. This information may include:

— an estimate of population size and trends of displacement;
— the rates and the major causes of mortality;
— the existence of diseases of epidemic potential, such as measles, cholera, and meningitis;
— the major causes of morbidity;
— the availability of food and the nutritional situation; and
— the population's basic environmental needs, such as water, shelter, and sanitation facilities.

A checklist will ensure that important data are not forgotten. The sample checklist on page 60 is provided as an example.

Assessing health status

Assessing health status consists of collecting demographic and background health information, and information on the three key indicators for a displaced population's state of health: nutritional status, mortality and morbidity.

Demographic characteristics

- The following information should be collected:
    — population size with age–sex breakdown (e.g. <1, 1–4, 5–14, 15–44, 45–59, >60 years old);
    — number of arrivals and departures per week;
    — predicted number of future arrivals;
    — ethnic composition and place of origin;

- identification of at-risk groups, (e.g. infants less than one year, children less than five years, pregnant and lactating women, households headed by women, unaccompanied children, disabled and wounded, elderly); and
  - average family or household size.
- This information is needed because:
  - the total population is the denominator for all death and morbidity rates, which might be estimated at later stages;
  - estimating population size makes calculating emergency supplies possible; and
  - a breakdown of the population by age and sex allows for the targeting of special interventions (e.g. immunization and care for pregnant and lactating women).
- Demographic information can be obtained from:
  - existing reliable census;
  - registration records maintained by camp administrators, local government officials, religious leaders, and others;
  - interviews with leaders within the displaced groups;
  - visual inspection during a walk through the area (This gives a quick impression of sanitary conditions and population density. Note, however, that it is unwise to base conclusions on visual impressions alone. Depending on the time of day and cultural habits, the population may differ. For instance, people may be gathering firewood away from the settlement);
  - aerial photography and use of global positioning systems (GPS); and
  - a small survey. (In sampled dwellings, record the number of family members, age and sex of each, and the number of pregnant and lactating women. Calculate the average number of persons per visited dwelling, then the total number of dwellings in the camp or settlement.)

Given that no rapid method is entirely reliable, a combination of them and comparison of the resulting estimates should be used. As soon as possible, ensure that a system for registering new arrivals is established. Record the names of household heads, number of family members by age and sex, former place and region of residence, and ethnic group, where applicable.

Background health information
- The following information should be collected:
  - main health, nutritional, and psychosocial problems in place of origin and among host population;
  - public health programme coverage in place of origin and among host population (e.g. measles immunization);
  - previous sources and types of health care, including traditional medicine;
  - availability of health workers in the displaced population;
  - important health beliefs and traditions; and
  - social organization.
- This information is needed in order to:
  - identify current health priorities for immediate intervention;
  - identify potential health threats;

- collect baseline information for future monitoring; and
- ensure appropriateness of planned health interventions.
- Background health information can be obtained from:
  - documents and reports from the host government ministry of health and universities, as well as international and nongovernmental organizations (collect information on endemic diseases and public health programmes in the displaced population's place of origin and in the host area);
  - interviews with community leaders, household heads, health workers, and individuals; and
  - development organizations, private companies, and missionaries with experience with the displaced population.

Nutritional status

- The following information should be collected:
  - prevalence of acute protein–energy malnutrition in children 6 to 59 months of age or 60 to 110 centimetres in height; and
  - prevalence of micronutrient deficiencies.
- This information is needed, in combination with information on food sources and security, to design feeding interventions and to identify groups at nutritional risk.
- Information on nutritional status can be obtained from:
  - anthropometric and micronutrient deficiency screening on all newly arrived children (or a sample of children if there are insufficient personnel, or too many new arrivals);
  - inclusion in any household survey of an assessment of nutritional status using anthropometric measures and micronutrient deficiency screening;
  - weight-for-height measurement[1] and examination for clinical signs of vitamin A, B and C deficiencies (see Chapter 8);
  - review of local hospital records (e.g. admissions and deaths due to malnutrition);
  - interviews with resource people among the displaced (assess food availability before displacement and the duration of the journey from place of origin to the present site); and
  - visual inspection, bearing in mind that it is unwise to base conclusions about childhood nutritional status on visual impressions alone.

Mortality

Death rates will be very difficult to calculate accurately in a rapid health assessment, owing to the lack of time for collecting and analysing information. Reliable death rates can be calculated only if:

- census information has already been systematically collected by national authorities or other organizations that provides a total population count by age and sex;
- the population remains static other than births and deaths (there are few people joining or leaving the population)·

[1] Mid-upper arm circumference (MUAC), and QUAC (MUAC for height) can also be used, but are considered less accurate than weight-for-height measures.

— a mortality surveillance system is in place;
— the information is classified appropriately, e.g. in rational age groups, independently for both sexes;
— mortality information is collected over a statistically valid period of time (where mortality is very high, this period can be quite short—where it is low, sporadic, or of uncertain causes, then this can be a very long period);
— death rates are calculated by a national demographer or, if a demographer is not available, an epidemiologist.

However, approximate death rates can still be estimated if only a few of these conditions are not present. It may be possible to calculate: crude death rate (number of deaths per 10 000 people a day), age-specific death rates (number of deaths per 10 000 people of a given age group per day), and cause-specific death rates (number of deaths from a given cause per 10 000 people a day).

- To calculate crude death rate, age-specific death rates, and cause-specific death rates, the following information should be collected:
  — population numbers by sex and by rational age groupings (e.g. <1, 1–4, 5–14, 15–44, 45–59, >60);
  — number of deaths over a statistically valid time period (crude death rate);
  — number of deaths for relevant age groupings over a statistically valid time period (age-specific death rates); and
  — number of deaths and the expected causes of each death over a statistically valid time period (cause-specific death rates).
- This information is needed because the crude death rate and the death rate in children less than five years of age are important overall indicators of the population's health. For any country in the world there is an estimate of the crude death rate available. This figure should be noted by the rapid assessment team, and compared with calculated death rates in given situations. Table 5 indicates the degree of severity of different death rates, although the actual figures are value judgements rather than scientific indicators.
- Information on mortality can be obtained from:
  — a system of mortality surveillance (a sample morbidity and mortality weekly surveillance form is shown on page 61);
  — designation of a single burial site for the camp or settlement, monitored by 24-hour grave-watchers, and development of a verbal autopsy procedure for expected causes of death using standard forms (Remember that death registration may be incomplete if rations are

Table 5. **Degree of severity of different death rates**

Degree of severity	Crude death rate (deaths/10 000/day)	Under-five death rate (deaths/10 000/day)
Normal or mildly elevated	0.3–1.0	0.6–2.0
Severe	1.0–2.0	2.0–4.0
Critical	>2.0	>4.0

reduced for a family after a death is reported, because of the desire to retain rations);
— hospital records and records of organizations responsible for burial;
— interviews with community leaders; and
— mandating registration of deaths, issuing shrouds to families of the deceased to help ensure compliance, monitoring records of private burial contractors, or employing volunteer community informants who report deaths for a defined section of the population (e.g. 50 families).

Morbidity
- The following information should be collected:
  — number of cases of various diseases, including diseases that cause substantial morbidity, such as diarrhoea, respiratory infections, and malaria, and diseases that may occur in large epidemics, such as measles, cholera, and meningitis; and
  — population size.
- Information on morbidity can be obtained from:
  — local hospital and clinic records;
  — patient registers and records in camp or settlement clinics, hospitals or feeding centres;
  — interviews with resource people within the displaced population (e.g. midwives and other health workers); and
  — a simple morbidity surveillance system. (When deciding whether a disease should be included in routine surveillance, consider the proportion of all morbidity caused by the disease, the seriousness of the disease in terms of the likelihood that it will result in death, and the likelihood that the disease will spread rapidly and result in a large epidemic.)

Assessing environmental conditions
Two priorities should be borne in mind in environmental assessment: shelter and water. Displaced persons can die quickly of exposure without shelter in inhospitable climates and within a few days without adequate water. To assist in setting priorities for public health programmes, information should be gathered on a number of elements.

Water supply
Information is needed on the current sources of water supply, the quantity, the quality, and the transport and storage capacity, including storage in households.

Sanitation
Information is needed on current methods of excreta disposal, the availability of soap, the presence of disease vectors, including rats, and the adequacy of burial sites.

Material possessions of displaced persons
Information is needed on the amount of blankets and clothing, shelter material, and domestic utensils (especially for preparing food and collecting water), as well as livestock, funds and other possessions.

Characteristics of the location

Information is needed on the following:

— climate, including seasonal variations;
— access to location by road, rail, and air;
— availability of land and extent of crowding;
— security against natural and man-made hazards;
— availability and proximity to building materials for shelter, and to fuel;
— soil topography and drainage; and
— possibility of foraging for foodstuffs.

Methods of collecting information

This assessment is largely carried out by visual inspection. Interviews with local officials and technical specialists are useful. In some instances, special surveys should be performed (e.g. investigations by entomologists for local disease vectors and water engineers to assess water resources).

Assessing local response capacity and immediate needs

Coordination

The information below should be obtained from national and international organizations, United Nations organizations, and NGOs working in the emergency-affected area:

• Who is in charge of coordinating health, water, and sanitation activities?
• Who supplies what services in these sectors?
• Who coordinates food delivery to the area and its distribution to the affected population?

Food supplies and sources

Well-nourished people can last days without food; however, already malnourished people may need food much sooner.

• Assess the quantity and type of food available to the population. If food is already being distributed, estimate the average number of calories received per capita for the period for which food distribution records are available.
• Assess the quality of the food available, its caloric and micronutrient content, and its acceptability to the recipient population.
• Inspect local markets for food availability and prices. Assess what foods are being traded and their exchange value.
• Assess local, regional, and national markets for availability of appropriate emergency foods.
• Include in any household survey an estimate of food stores in each household, looking for obvious inequalities between different families, ethnic or racial groups.
• Assess the cash and material resources of the displaced population to estimate their local purchasing power.

Feeding programmes

• Assess feeding programmes (general ration for the entire population, selective feeding for those at increased nutritional risk, and therapeutic

feeding for severely malnourished persons) set up by local officials, NGOs, church groups, local villagers, or other groups (see Chapter 8).
- A detailed assessment of feeding programmes could include admission criteria, figures for enrolment, attendance and discharge, quantity and quality of food provided, managerial competence, availability of water, utensils, and storage.

Health services and infrastructure

To assess health services and infrastructure available to the displaced population, the following should be considered.

- **Access**:
  — access by the displaced population to local pre-existing health facilities; and
  — ability of local health services to absorb the influx of displaced persons.
- **Facilities**:
  — type of facilities available, i.e. number of clinics, hospitals, and feeding centres;
  — size, capacity, and type of structures (tent, local materials, permanent structure) of health facilities set up specifically for displaced population; and
  — adequacy of health facilities' water supply, refrigeration facilities, and generators and fuel.
- **Personnel**:
  — type of health personnel and relevant skills and experience present in the hosting area (include sanitary experts, nutritionists, nurses, and doctors working in the private sector);
  — health workers present among the displaced population, including traditional healers, traditional midwives, doctors, and nurses; and
  — availability of interpreters.
- **Drugs and vaccines**:
  — availability of essential drugs and medical supplies; and
  — availability of essential vaccines and immunization equipment.
- **Non-food items**:
  — availability of items needed to address needs identified in the section above;
  — storage facilities for vaccines (cold chain), food, and non-food items; and
  — transport, fuel, and communications.

Presenting results

In presenting the results of your assessment, indicate the following information.

- Summarize rapid assessment findings, according to the headings listed in this document.
- Estimate, quantify, and prioritize needs for additional assistance, based on preliminary findings (e.g. food, drugs, technical personnel, equipment for improving water quality, and vector control measures).
- Prepare and convey assessment findings to appropriate emergency health decision-makers at subnational, national, and international levels.

Box 2. **Sample checklist for rapid health assessment in sudden population displacements**

Characteristics of the population and location

Demographic characteristics
- Total population size
- Proportion less than and greater than five years of age
- Size of at-risk groups
- Average household or family size

Background health information
- Main health and nutritional problems before displacement
- Coverage of public health programmes
- Previous sources of medical care
- Number and type of health workers in population
- Health beliefs and traditions
- Social organization

Nutrition
- Protein-energy malnutrition
- Micronutrient deficiencies

Mortality
- Crude death rate
- Age-specific death rates (less than and greater than five years of age)
- Cause-specific death rates

Morbidity
- Number of cases (and rates) of specific diseases

Water and sanitation
- Sources
- Quantity
- Quality
- Transport and storage
- Excreta practices
- Soap
- Vectors, including rats
- Burial sites

Material possessions
- Blankets and clothing
- Shelter
- Domestic utensils
- Livestock, money

Location
- Access
- Amount of land
- Other hazards
- Building materials and fuel
- Climate
- Topography and drainage

Response capacity
Coordination and services by existing organizations

Food available
- Access to local supplies
- Type of food
- Quantity
- Quality
- Feeding programmes

Health services available
- Access to and capacity of local services
- Health personnel
- Interpreters
- Type of facilities
- Type of structures
- Water, refrigeration, and generators at facilities
- Drug and vaccine supplies

Other materials available

Logistics
- Transport
- Fuel
- Storage of food, vaccines, and other supplies
- Communication

Box 3. **Sample morbidity and mortality weekly surveillance form**

This form should be adapted for specific situations.

From:____/____/____/ To:____/____/____/
Town/Village/Settlement/Camp:_____

Population

Population at beginning of week	
Births this week	+
Deaths this week	−
Arrivals this week	+
Departures this week	−
Estimated population at end of week	
Total population under five years of age	

Mortality

Reported primary cause of death	Female/age						Male/age						Total
	<1	1–4	5–14	15–44	44–59	>60	<1	1–4	5–14	15–44	44–59	>60	
diarrhoeal disease													
respiratory disease													
malnutrition													
malaria													
measles													
trauma													
other/unknown													
Total													

Average crude rates (deaths/10 000 total population/day)

Average under-five year old death rates (deaths/10 000 total under-fives/day)

Box 3. **Continued**

Morbidity

Primary symptom/ diagnosis	Female/age						Male/age						Total
	<1	1–4	5–14	15–44	44–59	>60	<1	1–4	5–14	15–44	44–59	>60	
diarrhoea/ dehydration													
fever with cough													
fever and chills/malaria													
measles													
trauma													
other/unknown													
Total													

Comments

_____

_____

_____

_____

Chapter 8
Nutritional emergencies

Purpose of assessment

The purpose of a rapid nutrition assessment is to:

— establish that a nutritional emergency or the risk of a nutritional emergency exists;
— identify the main causes of the emergency, estimate its severity and geographical extent;
— assess its likely evolution and impact on health and nutritional state;
— identify the areas and the socioeconomic groups most affected or at risk;
— assess existing response capacity and identify the most effective measures to prevent or minimize the nutritional emergency; and
— establish or expand existing surveillance, so that the effectiveness of measures taken can be monitored over time.

Background

The existence of a nutritional emergency should be considered whenever a population has reduced access to food, associated with actual or threatened increases in morbidity and mortality.

In most instances, a food emergency is not an acute event, but one that develops over time. Early signs ("leading indicators") such as decreased rainfall can appear before access to food is reduced. At a later stage, there are indications of diminished access to food (for example, low food supplies and an increase in prices: "intermediate indicators"). Actual weight loss, mortality, and population migration usually occur at a relatively late stage in a nutritional emergency ("trailing indicators").

For the rapid assessment to be useful in a response, it must be sensitive to the signs of the famine's various stages: for example, occurrence of precipitating factors, implementation of coping strategies, destitution, migration, and epidemic mortality and morbidity.

Patterns of work and climate such as exposure to cold also affect food requirements and related mortality, and should also be considered in the assessment.

Information on a potential nutritional emergency may come from a range of sources: a famine early warning system, health or other government officials, and nongovernmental organizations. Therefore, it is essential to carry out a rapid assessment to confirm or refute these initial reports.

The rapid assessment should not take longer than four to seven days. By comparison, a more thorough assessment requires between two and three weeks, because it includes large-scale, population-based surveys. It is most effectively carried out as a team effort, with specialists' input on food logistics, agriculture, and health.

Preparedness

This type of assessment must always be carried out, or at least closely supervised by a professional nutritionist, who should be identified in advance. Health workers should be routinely trained to carry out a rapid nutrition assessment according to standard guidelines which should be ready for use by all organizations. They should specify such information as anthropometric indicators, reference standards, cut-off points, and intervention criteria.

Essential equipment should be easily available (e.g. weighing scales, height boards, MUAC tapes, and pocket calculators).

Conducting the assessment

The rapid assessment consists of:

— confirming the first information (is there a nutritional emergency?);
— identifying the main causes;
— assessing the severity of the problem;
— identifying measures to minimize or prevent the emergency; and
— ensuring monitoring and surveillance.

Confirming the first information: is there a nutritional emergency?
Look for any of the signs listed below.

- Indications of ongoing nutritional emergency:
  — problems with access to food;
  — deteriorating nutritional status; and
  — obviously elevated mortality.
- Indications of nutritional risk:
  — rumours of famine and malnutrition;
  — drought or flooding;
  — information on excessive sale of animals, household items, and wood;
  — consumption of crisis food;
  — major pests affecting crops or livestock;
  — seasonal stress (e.g. pre-harvest gap, "lean season");
  — declining food stocks at household, district, and national levels;
  — rising market prices;
  — disruptive conflicts;
  — major displacements of population; and
  — history of previous famines.

Identifying the main causes

The points below should be considered when identifying the main causes:

— types and quantities of food available at household, community and district (or national) level;
— availability of staple foods in local markets and prices (What staple foods are available? Have prices increased or decreased or stayed the same?);
— current and predicted availability of local crops;
— existence and size of household food stores, household gardens;
— purchasing power (e.g. income from labour or sales of assets);
— employment;
— availability and cost of other key commodities (e.g. water, fuel);
— access to land;
— availability of seed, fertilizers, etc.;
— recent migrations (inwards, outwards);
— food distribution (how frequent, date of last distribution, how much food, estimated caloric content per person, what types?); and
— inaccessible areas, logistic bottlenecks.

Assessing the severity of the problem, the geographical extent, and the socioeconomic groups at risk

In making this assessment, the following information should be gathered:

— occurrence of epidemics or endemic diseases;
— coverage by health systems and programmes;
— environment, water, sanitation and food safety;
— patterns of settlement; displacement, shelter, and clothing;
— changes in work patterns and sources of household food supplies: percentage of household income being used on food; and
— signs of family disruption, violence, abandoned children and elderly, interruption of breast-feeding, and decrease in school attendance.

Assessing children's nutritional status

Increased mortality in nutritional emergencies is most likely related to malnutrition, an expected outcome of acute food deficits, communicable diseases, and environmental exposure. Because these effects are more readily detected in children, rates of acute or recent child malnutrition can be used to indicate mortality risk.

Clinical assessment

Always assess for kwashiorkor (oedema) which is classified as "severe malnutrition". If sufficient expertise is available, assess for signs of deficiency of vitamin A (xerophthalmia), B1 (beriberi), niacin (pellagra), iron, and other micronutrient deficiencies, as these frequently occur in famine-affected populations. These may require biochemical (laboratory) confirmation.

Anthropometric assessment

Child malnutrition can be most easily assessed by measuring weight-for-height, of a representative group of children. Mid-upper-arm-circumference (MUAC) and arm circumference for height (QUAC) can also be used. Weight-for-age should not be used because it may reflect the low height-for-age associated with chronic malnutrition.

Weight-for-height is used extensively and is more accepted as an indicator of acute malnutrition, but it requires both weight and length measurements, and the equipment is heavy.

Mid-upper-arm-circumference is quick to measure, relates well to mortality risk and is appropriate for identifying severely thin children. However, it is poorly related to weight-for-height, requires care in measurement, and is a poor tool for surveillance and monitoring of nutritional change over time.

Arm circumference for height directly relates to the nutritionally significant tissues, lean body mass, and fat mass. It is quick and easy to perform. It is usually parallel to weight-for-height but the correlation may vary according to ecological conditions.

Assess adult nutrition in a subsample

While assessing adult nutrition along with child nutrition is still not widely practised, it makes it possible to distinguish communities with an overall chronic dietary energy deficit (where generalized feeding is necessary) from ones in which only young children are affected. In the latter case the deficit may be due to widespread infections or to young child feeding practices (therefore, nutrition education is needed). Adult nutrition is measured in terms of the body mass index, i.e. weight in kilograms/(height in metres)^2. The accepted lower limit of normal in terms of the body mass index for adult men and women is 18.5.

Strategies for collection

Review existing data, consult hospital registers, etc. Interview community leaders, etc. (see Chapter 1).

One approach for gathering information is to carry out a nutrition survey of a sample of children between six months and five years of age (between 65 centimetres and 110 centimetres in height). Depending on the time available, and the size and dispersion of the population, this is also an opportunity to collect baseline data on immunization status and childhood mortality in the past month. Annex 2 shows reference values for rapid health assessment in developing countries.

Care should be taken when interpreting anthropometric survey findings. Although a malnutrition rate may be useful in confirming the severity of a food emergency, it must be complemented by other data (see above).

Assess child mortality and morbidity

Information on the recent mortality of young children (e.g. in the past month) is a useful indicator of the severity and duration of food shortfalls.

Mortality and morbidity information is also helpful for targeting immediate public health interventions. For instance, if deaths have been due to diarrhoea or measles, what proportion of mortality is in neonates?

Information on mortality and morbidity is essential for correct interpretation of the findings of a nutrition survey. If high mortality among nutritionally vulnerable children occurred in the preceding month(s), then it is quite possible that many of the more malnourished children have died and a low malnutrition prevalence will be observed in a survey of the survivors.

This information can be gathered from community leaders, burial records, and cemeteries, or collected during a survey of households.

Measuring the nutritional status of a population

Anthropometric surveys allow us to quantify the severity of the nutritional situation at one point in time, which is essential to help plan and initiate an appropriate response.

The prevalence of malnutrition in the 6–59-month age group is used as an indicator for nutritional status of the entire population, because:

— this subgroup is more sensitive to nutritional stress; and
— interventions are usually targeted to this group.

To ensure that the estimate will be representative of the whole population, random, systematic or cluster sampling procedures must be used.

During the survey, the nutritional status of individual children is assessed, prevalence of malnutrition is then expressed as the percentage of children moderately and severely acutely malnourished. It is very important to mention:

— the indicator (weight-for-height, oedema, MUAC, QUAC);
— the method of statistical description (% of the median, Z-score); and
— the cut-off points used.

Results should always be expressed as the percentage of children Z-score < -2 and Z-score < -3 and/or with oedema, to allow international comparisons as well as for statistical reasons.

However, it also might be necessary to express the results using a different classification system, if that is the method generally used in the area in which you are working.

The definitions of malnutrition for the different indicators are shown in Table 6.

The preferred method of assessment in children is by weight-for-height, and in adults by body mass index (see above).

Mid-upper-arm-circumference (MUAC) is an often-used anthropometric indicator. Formerly one cut-off level was considered usable for children aged from six or twelve months up to five years. But there is an average increase of about 3 centimetres in arm circumference over this time. WHO and the Centers for

Table 6. **Definitions of malnutrition**

	Malnutrition	*Moderate malnutrition*	*Severe malnutrition*
Children aged 0.0–59.9 months	WFH Z-score <−2 or <80% median WFH or MUAC <12.5 cm and/or nutritional oedema	WFH −3 ≤ Z-score <−2 or 70–79% median WFH or 11.0 cm ≤ MUAC <12.5 cm	WFH Z-score <−3 or <70% median WFH or MUAC <11.0 cm and/or nutritional oedema
Children aged 5.0–9.9 years	WFH Z-score <−2 or <80% median WFH and/or nutritional oedema	WFH −3 ≤ Z-score <−2 or 70–79% median WFH	WFH Z-score <−3 or <70% median WFH and/or nutritional oedema
Adults aged 20.0–59.9 years	BMI <17 and/or nutritional oedema	16 ≤ BMI <17	BMI <16

WFH = weight-for-height.
MUAC = mid-upper-arm circumference.
BMI = body mass index.

Disease Control and Prevention, Atlanta, USA, have prepared reference values for mid-upper-arm circumference for age, and also for height. In the field, it is sometimes difficult to determine age precisely and therefore determining approximate nutritional status by arm circumference for height is more feasible. A QUAC stick that gives reference values for arm circumference in terms of height is available for the management of nutrition in major emergencies.

However, the risk of measurement error is very high; therefore MUAC is used only for quick screening and rapid assessments of the nutritional situation of the population to determine the need for a proper weight-for-height random survey.

Assessing local response capacity

In order to respond promptly to food emergencies, it is important to identify local programmes and services that can be expanded quickly, and those technical, managerial and logistic gaps that need to be filled to support these efforts.

It is essential to identify a full range of response options, including supportive public health interventions, such as improved access to clean water and strategies that increase purchasing power if food is available but too costly for the affected population.

In many situations, a community will temporarily extend assistance to those who have migrated from other areas. The information collected should help guide the decision as to whether to extend food or other assistance to both settled and displaced populations, or to target only the displaced who can be expected to be the most vulnerable. Care should be taken to avoid discrepancies in food supply or access to health services between the displaced and settled host populations.

General response

A rapid assessment should gather at least enough information from the affected community to answer the following questions.

- Are the affected communities able to cope with their own resources, considering the access to food and the prevailing health situation?
- If not, what would be the possible interventions (for the immediate, medium, and long term)?
- What would be the key technical, managerial, logistic, and material requirements for each approach?
- What are the main constraints? What is needed to overcome them?
- What nutrition-supportive health measures should be implemented immediately?

Technical capacity

- What is the national-level capacity for deciding on food distribution requirements and rations?
- Are there experienced people locally available to carry out food distribution?
- Can health coverage be expanded to offset the increased hazards? Are there outpatient or mother and child health (MCH) clinics whose nutrition functions could be expanded?
- If so, are local health workers trained to detect and manage malnourished children, including those with important vitamin or mineral deficiencies?
- Are there trained health workers or traditional birth attendants who could take a role in ensuring MCH or nutrition coverage or both of the affected population?
- Is there a person or organization experienced in setting up MCH or nutrition outreach programmes or both in the past who could assist in establishing them in the affected communities?
- Is any selective feeding being undertaken? (Are guidelines being followed? What is the caloric content of meals provided?)

Availability of food stocks

- What is the food availability (amount and types) at central and subnational levels?
- Which food commodities are in the pipeline?

Logistics and managerial capacity

- What is the condition of road, rail, and boat access to the affected population (e.g. sealed roads, access in rainy season, air access, and security)?
- Are there facilities that could serve as warehouses? (What is the storage capacity? Is there adequate physical infrastructure?)
- What can be done to identify and register families in need of food assistance (e.g. through community leaders, church groups, and official registration procedures)?
- What access is there to radio communication between local, subnational, and central levels?

Public health response capacity
(See Chapter 7)

- Have the people left their home? Have they gathered in camps?
- How congested is the settlement? How many people per shelter?

- Is water available? In what quantity and quality? What is the source? How much does it cost?
- What are the sanitation arrangements?
- Are there trained water or sanitary engineers locally available?
- Where is the nearest vaccine store? Is it easily accessible? Are there trained vaccinators in the area? Is cold chain equipment available?

Identifying measures to minimize or prevent the emergency

Having identified the causes of the suspected famine, assessed its severity, and determined the local response capacity, it should be possible to identify measures to minimize or prevent the emergency.

- Determine the need for food distribution, e.g. what would be the type and quantity required for general or selective food distribution.
- Identify other non-ration options that would improve the nutritional status in areas where food is available but too costly for the population, e.g. create jobs through public works and improve access to water.
- Identify options for technical support (e.g. a qualified organization or individual to assist health workers in the affected population to improve the quality of selective feeding and early detection of malnourished children).
- Outline possible public health responses. These responses should benefit both the local population and possible displaced persons (e.g. by strengthening immunization and cold chain capacity of the affected area).

Ensuring monitoring and surveillance

It is necessary to ensure monitoring and surveillance of both the situation and any actions taken to remedy it.

- Collect information on existing systems for famine early warning, including nutritional status and epidemiological surveillance or surveys.
- Make recommendations for improvement ("filling the gaps").

In carrying out monitoring and surveillance, remember to:

— compare results of nutritional status surveys (using same criteria);
— look at data on nutritional deficiencies (morbidity data) in hospitals, health centres, and communities;
— monitor food distribution programmes, including number of calories per person per day (food basket surveys);
— monitor the number of admissions in the therapeutic feeding centre per week or month;
— monitor the percentage of children discharged from the therapeutic feeding centre: % of cured, % of dropouts, and % of deaths; and
— monitor the root causes identified by the assessment.

Implementing the selective feeding programme

Even if the overall food needs of a population are adequately met, inequities in the distribution system, disease, and other social factors may cause high degrees of malnutrition in certain vulnerable groups. Vulnerable groups may be targeted to receive a food supplement to upgrade their diet to a level that responds to their

Table 7 **Deciding on nutritional needs**

Finding	Action required
Food availability at household level below 2100 kcal (8.79 MJ)	Unsatisfactory situation • Improve general rations until local food availability and access can be made adequate.

Malnutrition rate[a] 15% or over
 	
or
 	
10–14% with aggravating factors[b]
	Serious situation
	• General rations (unless situation limited to vulnerable groups), plus:
	  – supplementary feeding generalized for all members of vulnerable groups (especially children, and pregnant and lactating women);
	  – therapeutic feeding programme for severely malnourished individuals.

Malnutrition rate[a] 10–14%
 	
or
 	
5–9% plus aggravating factors[b]
	Risky situation
	• No general rations, but:
	  – supplementary feeding targeted to individuals identified as malnourished in vulnerable groups;
	  – therapeutic feeding programme for severely malnourished individuals.

Malnutrition rate[a] under 10% with no aggravating factors[b]	Acceptable situation • No need for population interventions. • Attention to malnourished individuals through regular community services.

Notes
The above are only general indications. The best way to ensure that the nutritional needs of young children and other vulnerable groups are met is on a case-by-case basis, taking account of the particular local (including sociocultural) circumstances.
[a] Malnutrition rate: proportion of child population (aged six months to three or five years) who are below median -2 SD or 80% of reference value of weight-for-height.
[b] Aggravating factors:

— general food ration below the country-specific mean energy requirement;
— crude death rate >1 per 10 000 per day;
— epidemic of measles or whooping cough;
— high prevalence of respiratory or diarrhoeal diseases.

increased needs. Those that are already acutely malnourished must receive medical and nutritional attention to rehabilitate them to a healthy state. Table 7 can be used to help interpret the seriousness of the situation (it is intended as a guide, not as a set of rules).

Presenting results

In presenting the results of your assessment, indicate the following information:

Analysis and presentation of results

    — definition of population and areas affected and at risk;
    — identification of main causes;
    — information on current food access and projected food availability in the future;

— information on child and adult nutritional status, including micro-nutrient deficiencies;

— information on recent child mortality (including causes); and

— summary of existing response capacity, identifying gaps and possible areas to build on quickly, including immediate institutional strengthening and training.

Conclusions and recommendations

— possible response options, including food, water and sanitation measures, immunization and vitamin A distribution;

— recommended procedures for setting up health and nutrition surveillance of the at-risk populations and programme monitoring; and

— suggestions for further field investigations, to better estimate the size of the affected population, to improve possible targeting of food assistance, and to provide a better quality of baseline data for monitoring the effectiveness of response.

Chapter 9
Chemical emergencies

Purpose of assessment

The purpose of a rapid health assessment in a chemical emergency is to:

— confirm the existence of a chemical emergency;
— identify the characteristics of the chemicals involved as well as the source of release and estimate its type, size, location, and distribution;
— determine the population at risk and the impact on health; and
— assess local health response capacity.

Background

Most chemical accidents occur within the workplace, and may have no direct, large-scale or long-term effects. On such a limited scale, a rapid assessment is a relatively simple undertaking.

However, when a large number of people and a wider area are exposed to a chemical hazard, the assessment becomes a major exercise.

Most accidents occur at the interfaces between transport, storage, processing, use and disposal. This is where there are the fewest controls and the greatest probability of poor practices.

The risks of accidental chemical releases are greater with the number of new hazardous substances produced. First, production, storage, transport, and use of flammable, explosive or toxic chemicals have grown significantly in both developing and developed countries. Second, greater and more centralized productions have increased the quantities of chemicals manufactured and the distances they are transported. Third, population growth close to chemical plants and along transportation routes has meant that there are larger communities in greater number at high risk following a chemical accident.

The health impact of a chemical exposure is determined by the chemical itself, the exposure routes, and the amount of exposure. Exposure pathways vary, depending on the stage of the release. During the release, health effects from dermal exposure and inhalation can be expected. In the post-impact phase, the greater risks are dermal exposure, through contact with contaminated objects, and ingestion of contaminated food or water.

In many countries the ministry of health may not be responsible for managing chemical emergencies. However, the considerable health impact of a major chemical emergency calls for the active involvement of the health sector in the emergency preparedness process and in the assessment. The health sector should work closely with government agencies responsible for fire and rescue, paramedical services, security, environment, transport and dangerous goods.

Chemical incidents can cause an emergency:

— by acute release (e.g. exposure to corrosive effects of ammonia and gas used as refrigerant); and
— by chronic release (e.g. pyrrolizidine alkaloids found in plants that contaminate staple food crops and produce liver disease).

Also food contamination with chemicals or toxins can produce acute or slow onset emergencies that, either way, have long-term effects.

This protocol will focus on assessing an acute chemical release which requires an immediate response.

As discussed in Chapter 1, a chemical emergency should be first assessed within 24 hours following the incident at the latest. A more comprehensive assessment should be carried out later. Box 4 contains a sample checklist for rapid health assessment in chemical emergencies.

Conducting the assessment

The rapid assessment consists of:

— confirming the existence of a chemical emergency;
— determining the source, site, type, size and distribution of the release;
— identifying the specific types of chemicals and their reaction by-products;
— determining the population at risk and the health impact; and
— assessing existing health response capacity.

Confirming the existence of a chemical emergency

The first alert or rumour that a chemical emergency is occurring may originate from a wide range of sources. A quick visit to the site by a person with knowledge of handling dangerous goods or chemical expertise, taking suitable precautions, is important to verify this information.

The health personnel conducting the assessment should investigate the following questions:

• Has some incident happened involving chemical substances?
• Has some incident happened in or around a chemical installation?
• Has the community noted or have health facilities registered an increase in:
    — irritation of the eyes, the skin, the mucous membranes?
    — coughs, asthma, respiratory distress?
    — neurological illness?

Clinical examination of a sample of cases will help confirm the emergency.

Determining the source, site, type, size, and distribution of the release

This information is essential for defining the populations at risk, the potential range of exposures resulting from the accident, and the measures to be taken.

The exact site and type of incident should be determined, especially since a chemical emergency may involve one or more types of release. Other key characteristics include the size of the release (estimated weight or volume of the chemicals dispersed) and its distribution pattern (which is affected by weather conditions).

Identifying the types of chemicals and their reaction by-products

It is necessary to identify the chemicals involved in order to:

— anticipate their likely harmful effects;
— develop working case definitions of exposed and injured individuals and set criteria for triage;
— determine medical treatment for the injured and need for specific medication, decontamination, and follow-up regimens for those exposed;
— provide protective equipment for rescue personnel; and
— initiate control measures for environmental clean-up.

The identity, quantity, and ambient air concentrations of the chemical(s) can be determined through:

— product labels (product name, UN Hazard Classification and UN Substance Identification number);
— contacting companies in charge of the manufacture, storage, transport, use or disposal of the chemicals;
— contacting chemical information centres; and
— environmental sampling.

The collection of samples from the environment (air, water, food, soil, foliage) is important, since many unknown by-products may be produced in fires and explosions.

Determining the population at risk and the health impact

Determine the population at risk. Gather information on the proximity and size of residential neighbourhoods, the location and numbers of high-risk populations (e.g. individuals with chronic illnesses, pregnant women, and infants).

Evaluate toxicological risks and human exposure pathways. Environmental exposure and body burden assessments are usually not feasible during the acute phase of the accident. These require complex sampling and labour-intensive analytical procedures.

Describe morbidity and mortality. For this to be done systematically, it is essential that a working case definition is developed, and consistently applied. During the actual emergency, it is not feasible to conduct a survey. However, it is important to collect information on whether there has been increased morbidity or mortality caused by the release.

Analysing the information

Time: When did the cases occur? Is their number increasing?

- Plot the daily number of cases on a graph.
- If the chemical accident has affected a wide area, plot a separate graph for each affected community.
- Survey known exposed groups.

Place: Where have cases occurred? Are new cases being reported from other areas? Are there accessible, equipped, and safe health facilities in the affected areas?

- Map the cases geographically.
- Use maps that have health facilities identified.

Person: Which groups are at greatest risk?

- Examine data on age, sex, occupation, and residence to identify highest risk groups.
- Estimate the numbers of hospital admissions and outpatient attendances for affected areas and specific facilities.

Drawing initial conclusions

- Has a chemical release occurred?
- Has the causative chemical(s) been identified?
- What are the main risks for human health?
- How many cases or deaths so far?
- What is the geographical distribution of the cases?
- What is the size of the population at risk?
- Do the effects of the accident appear to be spreading?

Assessing local response capacity

The response capacity of health services should be assessed with particular attention to determine the following:

- availability of first-line and backup emergency medical services (including health personnel and facilities);
- availability of protective equipment;
- use of clear diagnostic criteria, standard treatment regimens, and compliance with them;
- availability of specific medication (e.g. antidotes);
- availability of facilities for decontaminating exposed individuals (including health workers); and
- vulnerability of the health facilities to the chemical.

Presenting results

In presenting the results of your assessment, indicate the following information.

- Define, quantify, and map the populations at risk or already affected by the release or both.

- Determine the likely health effects of the chemical release.
- Estimate the number of cases and deaths, and expected hospital admissions and outpatient attendances for the affected areas and specific facilities.
- Estimate needs for outside assistance, based on preliminary findings (e.g. qualified technical personnel, drugs, logistics, and communications support).

Give recommendations on:

— appropriate triage and case management;
— environmental control strategies to prevent further spread of chemical contaminants;
— the need for population evacuation and how to proceed: means of information and communication with community and relevant organizations, destination of evacuees, means of transport, and routes of evacuation;
— appropriate care for those evacuated to temporary shelters; and
— collection, identification, and management of dead victims.

Box 4. Sample checklist for rapid health assessment in chemical emergencies

The following checklist will be of value in assessing and reporting on chemical emergencies.

1. **General information**
1.1 date and time of the release
1.2 chemical released
1.3 location of the release
 — country
 — region
 — community
1.4 population centres closest to the release
1.5 time of the assessment

2. **Morbidity and mortality**
2.1 number of casualties
 — mildly affected
 — seriously affected
2.2 number of deaths

3. **Site of the release**
3.1 source
3.2 location of source and address
3.3 Are similar episodes being reported elsewhere?

4. **Type(s) of release (describe)**
4.1 atmospheric dispersion
4.2 explosion

4.3 fire
4.4 spill
4.5 other

5. **Size of release**
5.1 quantity of chemicals in the plant or storage site
 — weight (kilograms or tonnes)
 — volume (m^3 or litres)
5.2 amount of the leakage from a pipeline or a chemical tank (litres, tonnes or flow rate)

6. **Distribution of release**
6.1 meteorological conditions
 — temperature
 — wind direction
 — wind speed (metres per second)
 — rainfall
 — sunshine or cloud
 — weather stability
6.2 geographical characteristics
 — valleys
 — mountains

Box 4. **Continued**

— lakes, other waters
6.3 define risk zone
   — size (square kilometres)
   — area where personal
     protection is needed
   — type of protective clothes
     needed
   — type of respiratory protection

7. **Define the populations at risk**
7.1 number of individuals close to
   the release
7.2 number of individual houses
   close to the release
7.3 Are any of the following close to
   the release?
   — schools
   — day-care centres
   — hospitals
   — shopping centres
   — public buildings
   — other vulnerable sites
7.4 Is evacuation needed? If so,
   where?

8. **Identification of the
chemicals and their by-
products**
8.1 observations related to the
   release
   — colour
   — odour
   — signs and symptoms of
     exposed humans
   — signs of exposed animals
     and plants
   — other observations
8.2 information on the chemicals
   released
   — correct technical name
   — trade name(s) of the
     chemical(s)
   — generic name(s)
   — synonyms
   — UN number, Chemical
     Abstracts Service Registry
     number (CAS number)
   — placards (on vehicle)
   — UN hazard classification

— names of the by-products
— information source
   (individuals' names, chemical
   centres or written
   documents, data sheets)
8.3 environmental samples collected
   — what samples were collected
   — qualitative results of
     chemical analysis
     (chemicals identified)
   — quantitative results
     (concentration of chemicals
     in the environment)

9. **Toxicological evaluation**
9.1 safety information on the
   chemicals released
9.2 available information on the
   chemicals in databases and
   emergency response plan
9.3 physical and chemical properties
   of the chemicals
   — molecular formula (to be
     completed later)
   — molecular weight
   — conversion factor ($mg/m^3 =$
     x parts per million)
   — density
   — vapour pressure
   — boiling point
   — flammability point
   — critical temperature
   — explosiveness
   — solubility in water and other
     liquids
9.4 likely toxic effects of released
   chemicals
   — irritation
   — suffocation
   — chemical burns
   — dermal effects
   — effects on eyes
   — acute systemic effects
   — chronic effects
   — most critical health effects
   — significant concentrations in
     air may cause death, serious

Box 4. **Continued**

symptoms, mild symptoms, or no symptoms

9.5 likely exposure route
— inhalation
— dermal absorption
— ingestion (contaminated water, food)

9.6 sources of further information
— data sheets
— text books
— databases

9.7 possibilities for body burden measurement
— blood samples
— urine samples
— other samples

9.8 list of laboratories where analyses can be carried out
— names of laboratories, addresses, and phone numbers
— backup laboratories

10. **Appropriate treatment regimens**

10.1 describe (list) symptoms

10.2 describe standardized treatment
— maintenance of vital functions
— decontamination and enhancement of elimination
— general symptomatic treatment
— specific antidotes and their dose
— other specific poisoning treatment

10.3 psychological support (management of stress reaction)

10.4 registry of casualties

11. **Emergency medical care and health service needs and capabilities**

11.1 identify places where treatment can be given
— hospitals
— health centres
— field hospitals and temporary health centres
— public buildings (schools)

11.2 identify available human resources for therapy and first aid
— doctors
— nurses
— other health personnel
— volunteers

11.3 transport capabilities
— ambulances and other cars
— air transport capabilities
— transport routes available (map)

12. **Environmental health assessment**

12.1 water supply
— analysis of water safety for chemicals
— analysis of substitute water for chemicals and bacteria
— state of emergency water supply

12.2 food supply
— analysis of food contamination
— availability of safe food

12.3 suitable shelters

13. **General response operations**

13.1 overall command

13.2 sectors involved (e.g. police and fire brigade)

13.3 public information and communications
— awareness
— reassurance
— instructions

13.4 management of fatalities
— rescue operations for the dead
— morgue
— identification of dead victims
— burials.

Chapter 10
Complex emergencies

Purpose of assessment

The purpose of this type of rapid health assessment is to:

— assess the dynamics, magnitude, affected areas, and likely evolution of the emergency;
— assess the major health and nutritional impact of the emergency on the civilian population;
— identify groups and areas most at risk;
— assess existing response capacity and immediate needs in the health sector;
— identify short- and medium-term priorities for the delivery of health emergency response and recovery; and
— provide global indicators of life-threatening suffering to assist in mobilizing and managing humanitarian assistance.

Background

Complex emergencies are situations where "the cause of the emergency as well as the assistance to the afflicted are bound by intense levels of political considerations".[1]

Complex emergencies are characterized by varying degrees of instability and even collapse of national authority. This leads to loss of administrative control and to the inability to provide vital services and protection to the civilian population. One main feature of complex emergencies is the actual or potential generalized violence: against human beings, the environment, infrastructures, and property. Violence has a direct impact in terms of deaths, physical and psychological trauma, and disabilities. In conflicts characterized by rapidly shifting zones of combat, civilians often find themselves under crossfire. In many instances they become the primary targets of ethnic cleansing, murder, sexual violence, torture, and mutilation.

The other effects of conflict on public health are mediated by a variety of circumstances that include:

• Population displacement, with concentration in camps, public buildings or other settlements. This causes an increase in the risk of acute respiratory infections, diarrhoea and dysentery, measles and other epidemics. The

[1] *Coping with Major Emergencies — WHO Strategy and Approaches to Humanitarian Action.* Geneva, World Health Organization, 1995 (unpublished document WHO/EHA/95.1; available on request from the Division of Emergency and Humanitarian Action, World Health Organization, 1211 Geneva 27, Switzerland).

dependence on food rations entails a parallel and interacting risk of malnutrition and micronutrient deficiencies (see Chapter 7 and Chapter 8).

- The loss of opportunities and instruments of production, food stocks, and purchasing power, usually accompanied by the destruction of the commercial network can result in diffuse food shortages. In an effort to cope, the population may resort to migration, on an even larger scale than that directly caused by violence (see Chapter 8).
- Armed attacks and landmines, in addition to targeting the civilian population, can damage key infrastructures, such as roads, water plants, communications, and even health facilities.
- The general economic crisis brought on by decreased production, loss of capital, and increased military expenditure, can force cuts in the budgets for the social sectors.
- Insecurity and military operations may restrict access to large areas of territory and constrain the delivery of health services, as well as general response and recovery operations.

As a result of population displacement, economic disruption and widespread violence, access to health care and other vital resources decrease just when hazards and vulnerabilities increase. The effects of acute respiratory infection (ARI), diarrhoea, measles, and other epidemics are compounded by the collapse of health services, programmes for immunization, and disease control.

The overall outcome is a generalized increase in the risk of illness and death that extends beyond the immediate area of conflict, and severe, acute, and chronic psychological traumas. All this must be addressed through emergency and long-term interventions.

A final, major consideration is that health needs will increase as soon as the conflict subsides. Cease-fire may be accompanied by such operations as repatriating refugees and demobilizing soldiers, who will need special health programmes in the quartering areas, and demining, which demands special provisions for medical evacuation.

The health infrastructures, weakened by war and economic crisis, will face new demands for curative care, and a major backlog of preventive measures which could not be implemented for long periods (e.g. measles immunization). Population movements will increase greatly, while previously cut-off areas will suddenly become accessible. The health sector will be required to re-establish coverage, since equitable access to services will play a major role in stabilizing the community and contributing to the peace process.

Conducting the assessment

The assessment can be carried out either at national level, as in preparing a consolidated appeal for humanitarian assistance, or at subnational, provincial, district or local levels. With some differences, the categories of data needed for each level of assessment are the same: in Box 5 on p. 85 there is a form which has recently been used for rapid health assessment at local level in Bosnia and Herzegovina, and that can be adapted to other situations.

As the background explains, complex emergencies usually involve population displacement and at least the risk of famine. Therefore, this protocol is to be used in conjunction with Chapter 7 and Chapter 8.

Information can be collected from existing documents, interviews, visits to the affected areas (see Chapters 1, 7, and 8). The information collected from NGOs, the United Nations, other international organizations, and the media will be particularly relevant in complex emergencies.

The rapid assessment consists of: describing the conflict, the affected area and the population, assessing the health outcome, the specific variables, and existing resources and additional immediate needs.

Describing the conflict, the affected area, and the population

To put health needs in perspective within the context of complex emergencies, information about the following is needed:

— duration of the conflict;
— state and progress of political negotiations (e.g. discussions for cease-fire);
— patterns of violence;
— accessible population;
— inaccessible population;
— inaccessible areas;
— occurrence of epidemics;
— occurrence of starvation; and
— general economic situation.

Assessing the health outcome

This is done by looking at crude and under-five mortality rates and causes, cause-specific morbidity and acute malnutrition rates, at least for the most severely affected areas or groups.

Assessing the variables

Information on the following points will help identify priorities and outline programmes for intervention in the short and medium term.

Violence and security

Information should be collected on:

— deaths and injuries from violence;
— deaths and injuries from landmines;
— occurrence of sexual violence;
— occurrence of torture;
— attacks on health personnel and response and recovery operators;

— attacks on health facilities; number and percentage of health facilities destroyed, closed or inaccessible;
— attacks on water systems;
— attacks on agriculture, food-processing, storage and distribution systems;
— attacks on response and recovery convoys;
— attacks on other lifeline systems: electricity, public transport, communications; and
— use of other inhumane weapons (e.g. biological and chemical).

Population displacement

Information should be collected on occurrence and numbers involved (see Chapter 7):

— internally displaced persons (IDPs);
— refugees in neighbouring countries;
— actual and expected movements (voluntary repatriations, foreseen returns);
— unaccompanied children;
— existence of IDP camps; and
— concentrations in urban areas (e.g. rates of urban growth).

Loss of production, food stocks, purchasing power, and commerce

Information should be collected on the loss of production, stocks of food, purchasing power and commerce (see Chapter 8).

Assessing local response capacity and immediate needs

Local response capacity and immediate needs should be assessed to determine the type and quality of external support required. As far as possible this information should be collected by province or district (see Chapter 7).

Health networks and programmes

The following information should be gathered on health networks and programmes:

— national health strategies addressing the emergency;
— percentage of working health facilities;
— geographical distribution of national health personnel (are they also displaced?);
— function of health information system (at least epidemiological and nutritional surveillance);
— availability and performance of primary health care services and programmes;
— capacities for surgery and trauma care;
— state of blood bank and transfusion safety;
— national and international organizations and NGOs: health projects and areas of coverage;
— military health assets (as far as possible, of all conflicting parties);
— sectoral coordination mechanisms;
— health training activities;
— salaries of national health personnel;

— share of state budget allocated to health; and
— international assistance to the health sector.

Environment and infrastructure
Information should be collected on the following:

— susceptibility to (history of) natural technological hazards;
— percentage of functioning water systems (urban, rural, IDP camps);
— percentage of working sanitation systems (urban, rural, IDP camps);
— state of roads, bridges, airports, etc.;
— percentage of buildings destroyed, public and private;
— presence of unexploded landmines and ordnance;
— geographical and climatic features; and
— prevalence of endemic diseases, vectors, etc.

Humanitarian assistance
The following points should be considered when assessing the humanitarian assistance being offered and planning for future provision of humanitarian assistance:

— composition of humanitarian assistance package (food and non-food);
— special humanitarian assistance programmes (demobilization, mine-awareness, and demining);
— access to the territory (road convoys, river and sea shipping, airlifts and airdrops, "humanitarian corridors", "windows of peace", etc.);
— patterns of aid distribution (i.e. by government, NGOs, the United Nations), timetable, coverage and logistic network;
— communication network;
— security requirements and assets;
— coordination mechanisms;
— procedures for international aid agreements;
— rights and authorizations for movements of people and goods (overflight, transit, landing);
— customs regulations, clearance, and waivers;
— mobilization of resources (projects, appeals, and donors' response); and
— general budget for humanitarian assistance (at least data from latest appeal and, if possible, trends).

Presenting results

Consolidate the information and present a report that provides the following:

— a brief description, including the percentage of the population and territory directly affected by the conflict;
— selected indicators, to show the emergency's direct impact (e.g. mortality rates, number of displaced, extent of malnutrition, damage to infrastructure and economy);
— indicators showing the secondary impact of the emergency (e.g. increase in risk of illness and death by epidemic or endemic diseases or both);

— data on the damage suffered by the health sector (percentage of lost infrastructure and personnel, disruption of primary health care programmes, priority shortages in drugs or vaccines); and
— the coverage, constraints and coordination of response and recovery operations.

In the report, try to describe worst-case and best-case scenarios for the next 6–12 months. What will be the health priorities if the conflict continues or if a cease-fire or peace is reached? Make recommendations, highlighting:

— immediate and medium-term priorities for action in the health sector, and needs, as arising from the above; and
— the best approaches and strategies considering the situation and current humanitarian action.

During a complex emergency, the situation can change very rapidly. Therefore, it is necessary to be cautious about long-term assumptions, to carry out planned actions quickly, before the situation changes, and to report on the situation and actions at frequent intervals.

Box 5. **Sample form for rapid health assessment in complex emergencies**

Area: _____ Surrounding towns: _____

Date: _____ Assessor: _____

Background
Total population – current: _____ pre-war: _____

Age and sex distribution:

• population under five years
• other vulnerable groups?

Weather – current: _____ projected: _____

Who is in charge? _____

Food and agriculture
What are people eating now? _____

Source(s) of food: _____

Date of last air drop: _____

How is air drop, humanitarian aid distributed? _____

Does it reach those most in need? _____

Box 5. **Continued**

Market availability (and prices), include black market if possible: _____

_____

_____

Visual assessment of livestock: _____

Assessment of cooking fuel: _____

_____

Any seeds available for planting: _____

Overall assessment of food availability and needs – include timeframe for seeds, etc.

Health and nutrition
Who is in charge? _____

What health services exist? _____

Assessment of damage to health infrastructure:

_____

What public health programmes (vaccination, etc.) currently operate?

_____

Assessment of recent mortality (rates and causes):

_____

Assessment of recent morbidity (rates and causes):

_____

Evidence of epidemics: _____

(specifically check for measles, hepatitis, diarrhoea)

Current staff: _____

Current drug supplies: _____

Current medical supplies: _____

Box 5. **Continued**

Evidence of malnutrition: _____

Evidence of micronutrient deficiencies: _____

Particularly vulnerable groups: _____

Overall health assessment – include priorities for assistance:

Water and sanitation
Who is in charge? _____

Normal sources of water: _____

Current sources – for drinking: _____

for washing, etc.: _____ _____

Estimates of current quantities provided: _____

Is water tested or treated in any way? _____

If so, how? _____

Assessment of damage to water system: _____

Assessment of damage to sewer system: _____

Changes in water supply expected due to seasonal variation: _____

Assessment of solid waste disposal: _____

Problems with rat control: _____

Overall assessment: water supplies are adequate or inadequate; safe or unsafe?

Priorities for assistance: _____

Shelter and household function
Who is in charge? _____

Assessment of damage to housing: _____

Availability of construction materials, plastic, etc.: _____

What type of clothing are people wearing? _____

Availability of blankets, sleeping bags, etc.: _____

Box 5. **Continued**

Impact of upcoming weather or season: _____

Logistics and security
Who is in charge? _____

Possible routes for humanitarian assistance: _____

Assessment of roads and bridges, etc.: _____

Availability of local storage facilities: _____

Security_____

    – checkpoints: _____

    – local security: _____

Overall assessment: _____

Overall: Top priorities, constraints, etc.

Selected further reading

Amartya Sen. *Poverty and famines: an essay on entitlement and deprivation.* Oxford, Clarendon Press, 1981.

APELL: Awareness and Preparedness for Emergencies at Local Level: a process for responding to technological accidents. Paris, United Nations Environment Programme, Industry and Environment Programme Activity Centre, 1988.

Assessing needs in the health sector after floods and hurricanes. Washington, DC, Pan American Health Organization, 1987 (PAHO Technical Paper No. 11).

Bailey KV, Ferro-Luzzi A. Use of body mass index of adults in assessing individual and community nutritional status. *Bulletin of the World Health Organization,* 1995, 73(5):673–680.

Baltazar JC. The potential of the case-control method for rapid epidemiological assessment. *World health statistics quarterly,* 1991, 44(3):140–144.

Bennett S et al. A computer simulation of household sampling schemes for health surveys in developing countries. *International journal of epidemiology,* 1994, 23(6):1282–1291.

Brogan D et al. Increasing the accuracy of the Expanded Programme on Immunization's cluster survey design. *Annals of epidemiology,* 1994, 4(4): 302–311.

Control of epidemic meningococcal disease: WHO practical guidelines. Lyon, Fondation Marcel Mérieux, 1995.

Coping with stress in crisis situations. Geneva, United Nations High Commissioner for Refugees, 1992.

Devianayagam N, Nedunchelian K. Rapid epidemiologic assessment (editorial). *Indian pediatrics,* 1991, 28(5):459–462.

De Ville de Goyet C, Seaman J, Geijer U. *The management of nutritional emergencies in large populations.* Geneva, World Health Organization, 1978.

Disaster assessment: the weak link in international relief efforts. *Bulletin of the Pan American Health Organization,* 1985, 19(1):97–99.

Field guide on rapid nutritional assessment in emergencies. Alexandria, WHO Regional Office for the Eastern Mediterranean, 1995.

Guha-Sapir D. Rapid assessment of health needs in mass emergencies: review of current concepts and methods. *World health statistics quarterly,* 1991, 44(3):171–181.

Guidelines for cholera control. Geneva, World Health Organization, 1993.

Guidelines for evaluation and care of victims of trauma and violence. Geneva, United Nations High Commissioner for Refugees, 1993.

Guidelines for the control of epidemics due to Shigella dysenteriae type 01. Geneva, World Health Organization, 1995 (unpublished document WHO/CDR/95.4; available on request from Division of Child Health and Development, World Health Organization, 1211 Geneva 27, Switzerland).

Guidelines on security incidents. Geneva, United Nations High Commissioner for Refugees, 1992.

Handbook for emergencies. Geneva, United Nations High Commissioner for Refugees, 1982.

Harrison GA, ed. *Famine.* Oxford, Oxford University Press, 1988 (Biosocial Society Series, No. 1).

Health aspects of chemical accidents. Geneva, United Nations Environment Programme, 1994 (UNEP IE/PAC Technical Report No. 19).

Hlady WG et al. Use of a modified cluster sampling method to perform rapid needs assessment after Hurricane Andrew. *Annals of emergency medicine,* 1994, 23(4):719–725.

Lee HW, Dalrymple JM, eds. *Manual of hemorrhagic fever with renal syndrome.* Seoul, WHO Collaborating Centre for Virus Reference and Research, 1989.

Lillibridge SR, Noji EK, Burkle FM Jr. Disaster assessment: the emergency health evaluation of a population affected by a disaster. *Annals of emergency medicine,* 1993, 22(11):1715–1720.

Management of severe malnutrition: a manual for physicians and other senior health workers. Geneva, World Health Organization, 1998.

Mason JB et al. *Nutritional surveillance.* Geneva, World Health Organization, 1984.

Mental health of refugees. Geneva, World Health Organization, 1996.

Nutrition guidelines. Paris, Médecins Sans Frontières, 1995.

Nutrition in times of disaster. Report of an international conference, Geneva, September 27–30, 1988. Washington, DC, United States Agency for International Development, 1989.

Pearson R. Rapid assessment procedures are changing the way UNICEF evaluates its projects. *Hygie,* 1989, 8(4):23–25.

Physical status: the use and interpretation of anthropometry. Geneva, World Health Organization, 1995 (WHO Technical Report Series, No. 854).

Prevention and control of yellow fever in Africa. Geneva, World Health Organization, 1986.

Psychosocial consequences of disasters: prevention and management. Geneva, World Health Organization, 1992 (unpublished document WHO/MNH/PSF/91.3; available on request from Division of Mental Health and Prevention of Substance Abuse, World Health Organization, 1211 Geneva 27, Switzerland).

Public health action in emergencies caused by epidemics. Geneva, World Health Organization, 1986.

Recommendations on the transport of dangerous goods, 7th ed. New York, United Nations, 1991.

Sexual violence against refugees: guidelines on prevention and response. Geneva, United Nations High Commissioner for Refugees, 1995.

Smith GS. Development of rapid epidemiologic assessment methods to evaluate health status and delivery of health services. *International journal of epidemiology*, 1989, 18:S2–15.

Storage of hazardous materials. Paris, United Nations Environment Programme, Industry and Environment Programme Activity Centre, 1990 (UNEP IE/PAC Technical Report Series, No. 3).

Tessier SF, Durandin F. Use and limits of anthropometric indicators in emergency assessment of famine situations: an example from northern Uganda (letter). *Journal of tropical pediatrics*, 1989, 35(5):267–269.

The management and prevention of diarrhoea: practical guidelines. Geneva, World Health Organization, 1993.

The management of bloody diarrhoea in young children. Geneva, World Health Organization, 1994 (unpublished document WHO/CDD/94.49; available on request from Division of Child Health and Development, World Health Organization, 1211 Geneva 27, Switzerland).

The public health consequences of disasters. Atlanta, GA, Centers for Disease Control and Prevention, 1989.

The treatment of diarrhoea: a manual for physicians and other senior health workers. Geneva, World Health Organization, 1995 (unpublished document WHO/CDR/95.3; available on request from Division of Child Health and Development, World Health Organization, 1211 Geneva 27, Switzerland).

Uligaszek SJ, Welsby SM. A rapid appraisal of the nutritional status of Irian Jaya refugees and Papua New Guineans undergoing severe food shortage in the North Fly region. *Papua New Guinea medical journal*, 1985, 28(2):109–114.

United Nations Disaster Management Training Programme. *An overview of disaster management*, 2nd ed. Madison, WI, University of Wisconsin, 1992.

Use and interpretation of anthropometric indicators of nutritional status. *Bulletin of the World Health Organization*, 1986, 64(6):929–941.

Working Group on Viral Haemorrhagic Fever and Viral Neurological Diseases, Seoul, Republic of Korea, 24–26 August 1987 (report). Manila, WHO Regional Office for the Western Pacific, 1988.

Annex 1

Techniques for surveys during rapid assessment

The use of informal household surveys for rapid health assessment

Although large household surveys are time-consuming exercises, smaller surveys can be carried out more quickly in emergencies. During the initial assessment of an emergency, limited surveys using non-probability sampling of affected populations may provide an estimate of the extent of damage and immediate health needs for guiding emergency decisions. However, the results of these surveys may be difficult to compare to those of subsequent, more statistically valid ones.

Larger, statistically valid household surveys are a valuable tool during later stages of the emergency, when there is more time available to refine the initial estimates, based on the rapid health assessment. Given the variety of situations in which rapid household surveys may be conducted, each one must be designed specifically. This annex does not provide assistance in deciding what information to collect, writing interview questions, choosing a representative sample, and analysing the resulting data, all of which require skilled personnel. It does give a broad overview of some issues involved in conducting surveys during rapid health assessment.

The process of selecting a sample

The purpose of conducting a survey is to describe key characteristics of the population under study, such as the proportion of houses damaged by an earthquake or the proportion of children vaccinated against measles. To derive an accurate estimate, the survey sample must be representative of the overall population. Therefore, if the affected population is very large or dispersed over a large area, the survey sample should be taken from as wide an area as is practical and not restricted to a small sub-area, which may not be typical of the population as a whole. Moreover, surveys should avoid sampling only the most accessible members of the affected population (e.g. those living along roads, near markets or in the centre of town).

The first step of any survey is to define the area under study. It is usually best to draw a rough map of the area that would include as much detail as possible about where people live, relative population concentrations, and major geographical features, such as roads and rivers. Use local informants to provide overall information about an area, as well as information on which areas are most and least affected. Investigators may wish to draw their sample from areas showing a wide range of severity of impact. It is a good idea to ask different people their opinion. The next step is to decide how to select the sample and its size. This decision depends on a number of factors including:

— the size of the area under study;
— the number of investigators available;
— the amount of time available for the survey;
— the availability of transport;
— the distribution of the affected population (e.g. isolated households, villages, and camps); and
— the different circumstances facing people in various parts of the emergency-affected area.

The simplest and quickest survey can be done by choosing a sample of 50 households at random. Data collection in this survey may take two or three people only one afternoon or less to complete. More extensive surveys may be necessary, but will require more people and time to complete.

Cluster sampling is a technique developed to save on survey costs. It involves selecting random starting points and then subsequently choosing systematically. For example, in a rural area, 30 villages are chosen randomly from a list of all the villages in the affected area. Then in each village, a house is chosen at random and subsequent houses chosen by selecting the houses closest to that house. To select households spread over a larger area of the village, the team may choose to select every fifth or every tenth house until the required number of houses in that village is surveyed.

The number of households visited in each cluster depends on what is to be assessed. In the standard cluster survey used to assess vaccination levels, seven households are chosen in each cluster. Such a survey may require three to five teams of interviewers and take three days or more to complete. In some assessments, as many as 700 children must be found to estimate health parameters with the necessary degree of precision. Depending on the amount of travel needed, these surveys may require 10 or more teams and more than a week to complete. These large surveys may not be appropriate for rapid health assessment in sudden emergencies, such as natural emergencies or sudden population displacement, where information about the population is needed very quickly.

Annex 2

List of reference values for rapid health assessment in developing countries

1. General	
Cut-off values for emergency warning Health status	**More than**
• daily crude death rate	1/10 000 population
• daily under-5 death rate	2/10 000 children under 5
Nutrition status	
• acute malnutrition (weight-for-height $<-2Z$ scores) in under-5s	10% of children under 5
• growth faltering rate in under-5s	30% of monitored children
• low weight at birth (less than 2.5 kg)	7% of live births
Standard structure of population	**Average in the population**
• 0–1 year	4%
• 0–5 years	18%
• fertile women	24%
• pregnant women	5%
• expected births	4.4 per 100 population per year

2. Vital needs		
Water	**Indicator**	**Average requirement**
• quantity	no. of litres/person/day	20 litres/person/day
• quality	no. of users/water point	200 people/water point
(1 cubic metre = 1 tonne = 1000 litres)		(not more than 100 metres from housing)
Food	**kcal (MJ) content**	**Ration, kg/person/month**
• cereals	350 (1.46)/100 g	10.5
• pulses	335 (1.40)/100 g	1.8
• oil	860 (3.59)/100 g	1.2
• sugar	400 (1.67)/100 g	1.2
kcal value of recommended ration, person/day: Total kg/person/month for feeding		2100 kcal (8.79 MJ) 14.7 kg

Sanitation
Latrine: ideally one per family; minimum, one seat per 20 people (6–50 m from housing)
Refuse disposal: one communal pit (2 m × 5 m × 2 m) per 500 people

Household fuel	**Average need**
Firewood	15 kg/household/day
Note: with one economic stove per family, the needs may be reduced:	5 kg/stove/day

Space for accommodation	
• Individual requirements (shelter only)	4 m^2/person
• Collective requirements, including shelter, sanitation, services, community activities, warehousing and access	30 m^2/person

3. Health needs and care

Prevalent health hazards	**Expected attack rate in emergency situations**
• Acute respiratory infections in children under 5	10%/month in cold weather
• Diarrhoeal diseases in children under 5 (other than dysentery and cholera)	50%/month
• Malaria, in total non-immune population	50%/month

Essential primary health care activities	**Target**	**Optimal coverage of target**
• under-5 clinic and growth monitoring	all children of 0–59 months	100% of under-5s per month
• antenatal clinic	all pregnancies	50% of pregnancies per month
• tetanus toxoid	all pregnancies	30% of pregnancies per month
• assisted deliveries	all deliveries	1/12 of total annual deliveries per month
• BCG	all new births	1/12 of total annual births per month
• DTP1–TT1	all children 0–1 year	1/12 of total group per month
• DTP2–TT2	all children 0–1 year	1/12 of total group per month
• DTP3	all children 0–1 year	1/12 of total group per month
• Measles	all children 9–12 months	1/12 of total group per month
• STD/HIV prevention (by condoms)	all sexually active males	12 condoms per man per month

Health personnel requirements	**Output of one person/hour of work**
Activity	
• vaccination	30 vaccinations
• under-5 clinic and growth monitoring	10 children
• antenatal clinic	6 women
• assisted delivery	1 delivery
• outpatient department consultation	6 consultations
• outpatient department treatment (dressings, etc.)	6 treatments
Note: one person/day = 7 hours of field work	
Health workers emergency requirements (e.g. refugee camp) for vaccinations, growth monitoring, antenatal clinic, assisted delivery, outpatient department consultations and treatments, registry and clerical duties	60 staff × 10 000 population

Health supplies requirements	Needed
Essential drugs and medical equipment	
• The WHO emergency health kit	1 kit for 10 000 population/3 months
Nutritional rehabilitation	**Needs of each under-5 patient**
• oil	90 g/day
• milk	120 g/day
• sugar	70 g/day
Safe drinking-water	amount
a) to prepare 1 litre of stock solution 1%:	use 1 litre of water, plus:
	15 g calcium hypochlorite 70%
	or 33 g bleaching powder[a] 30%
	or 250 ml sodium hypochlorite 5%
	or 110 ml sodium hypochlorite 10%
b) to disinfect drinking-water with the stock solution:	use 0.6 ml or three drops of solution per litre of water;
	use 60 ml of solution per 100 litres of water.

(*Note:* allow the chlorinated water to stand at least 30 minutes before using)

4. Needs for epidemic response

• Cholera

Likely maximum attack rate	6% over 4 months
100% cases needing ORS	6.5 packets/patient
20% cases needing IV fluids	3 litres/patient
20% cases needing antibiotics: doxycycline 300 mg, 1 dose	1 tab per course

• Meningococcal meningitis

100% cases treated with oily suspension chloramphenicol	6 amps per course
100% population to be vaccinated	1 dose/person

• Measles

Likely maximum attack rate in non-immunized under-12s	10%
100% non-immunized under-12s to be vaccinated	1 dose/child
100% under-12s to be given vitamin A • children 6 months to 1 year	100 000 IU/child
• children 1 year and over	200 000 IU/child

• Typhus

100% population to be deloused		
Individual spraying with permethrin 1%	• adult	30 g
	• infant and child	15 g

5. Essentials of logistics

Weights and volumes

• Food	individual ration per month	14.7 kg
	amount per 10 000 people per week	36.8 tonnes

(1 tonne of food grains/beans in standard 50 kg bags occupies 2 m^3)

• Drugs and supplies:	1 WHO emergency health kit	860 kg, 4 m^3

---

[a] Chlorinated lime or bleaching powder is a white powder which is a mixture of calcium hydroxide, calcium chloride and calcium hypochlorite. It typically contains 20–35% available chlorine.

- Vaccines: 1000 doses of measles 3 litres
  1000 doses of DTP 2.5 litres
  1000 doses of BCG 1 litre
  1000 doses of polio 1.5 litres
  1000 doses of tetanus 2.5 litres
- Food for therapeutic feeding: standard under-5 patient 2 kg/week
  ration
- Family-size tents: 35–60 kg unit 1 tonne, 4.5 m^3
- Blankets compressed 1 tonne, 4.5 m^3
  loose 1 tonne, 9 m^3

Warehouse requirements	• approximately 25 m^2 for 1000 population
	• 1.2 m^2 for 1 tonne of bagged food grains stacked 6 m high
Average truck capacity	• 50 tonnes
Small aircraft capacity	• 3 tonnes

Sources: WHO/EHA, UNHCR Emergency Tools Series, draft 1992; UNICEF *Assisting in Emergencies*, 1986